STAY YOUNG

BY JOGGING

The Essential Fitness Guide for Life at age 40 and Beyond

Jeanelle K. Douglas

Contents

INTRODUCTION

Embarking on a jogging journey at the age of 40 marks a significant milestone in your fitness and wellness journey. While some may perceive age as a barrier to physical activity, it can, in fact, be the perfect time to embrace the rejuvenating benefits of jogging. Whether you're looking to boost your cardiovascular health, shed a few pounds, or simply enjoy the invigorating outdoors, jogging offers a plethora of advantages for individuals in their 40s and beyond.

In this guide, we'll explore the various aspects of starting jogging at 40, addressing both the physical and mental aspects of this endeavor. From assessing your current fitness level to creating a tailored jogging plan, we'll provide you with the tools and knowledge needed to embark on this fulfilling journey safely and effectively.

We understand that starting any new fitness routine can be daunting, especially as we age. That's why we're here to guide you through every step of the process, offering practical advice, tips, and motivation to help you overcome any obstacles along the way. Whether you're a complete novice or someone returning to jogging after a hiatus, this guide is designed to support you in achieving your health and wellness goals.

So lace up your shoes, step outside, and let's begin this exhilarating journey together. Whether you're jogging for the physical benefits, the mental clarity, or simply the joy of movement, you're taking a proactive step towards a healthier, happier you.

Let's make every stride count!!!

Why Jogging?

Jogging isn't just about putting one foot in front of the other, it's a transformative activity that can positively impact every aspect of your life.

Here are several compelling reasons why jogging at the age of 40 can be an incredibly rewarding pursuit:

1. Improved Cardiovascular Health: Jogging is one of the most effective cardiovascular exercises, helping to strengthen your heart and improve circulation. By getting your heart pumping and blood flowing, jogging can reduce the risk of heart disease, stroke, and high blood pressure.

2. Weight Management: As we age, our metabolism tends to slow down, making weight management more challenging. Jogging is a calorie-burning activity that can help you maintain a healthy weight or shed excess pounds. It's a fantastic way to boost your metabolism and burn calories both during and after your run.

3. Enhanced Mental Well-Being: The benefits of jogging extend beyond the physical realm, they can also positively impact your mental health. Jogging releases endorphins, often referred to as "feel-good" hormones, which can alleviate stress, anxiety, and depression. It provides an opportunity to clear your mind, reduce tension, and improve overall mood.

4. Increased Energy Levels: Contrary to common belief, regular exercise, such as jogging, can actually increase your energy levels. By improving circulation and oxygen flow throughout your body, jogging can boost your stamina and combat feelings of fatigue and lethargy.

5. Bone and Joint Health: Concerns about joint health are common as we age, but jogging can actually help strengthen bones and joints when done correctly. Weight-bearing exercises like jogging stimulate bone growth and improve joint flexibility, reducing the risk of osteoporosis and arthritis.

6. Improved Sleep Quality: Getting enough quality sleep becomes increasingly important as we age, and jogging can help you achieve just that. Regular physical activity, including jogging, can regulate your sleep patterns, making it easier to fall asleep and stay asleep throughout the night.

7. Sense of Achievement and Empowerment: Starting a jogging routine at 40 can instill a sense of accomplishment and empowerment. It's a tangible way to take control of your health and fitness, setting and achieving goals that boost your confidence and self-esteem.

In essence, jogging at 40 offers a myriad of physical, mental, and emotional benefits that can enhance your overall quality of life. It's a simple yet powerful activity that has the potential to transform your well-being for the better.

So why jog?

Because with each stride, you're not just moving forward physically, you're moving towards a healthier, happier you.

Benefits of Jogging at 40

1. Improved Cardiovascular Health: Jogging strengthens the heart and improves circulation, reducing the risk of heart disease, stroke, and high blood pressure. At age 40, maintaining cardiovascular health becomes increasingly important, and jogging is an effective way to achieve this.

2. Weight Management: Metabolism tends to slow down with age, making weight management more challenging. Jogging helps burn calories, boost metabolism, and maintain a healthy weight, combating age-related weight gain and promoting a leaner physique.

3. Enhanced Mental Well-Being: Jogging releases endorphins, which can alleviate stress, anxiety, and depression. At age 40, managing mental health becomes crucial, and jogging provides an outlet to clear the mind, reduce tension, and improve overall mood.

4. Increased Energy Levels: Regular jogging boosts stamina and combats feelings of fatigue and lethargy, providing a natural energy boost. This is particularly beneficial at age 40 when energy levels may start to decline, helping you stay active and engaged throughout the day.

5. Bone and Joint Health: Concerns about bone and joint health become more prevalent with age, but jogging can help strengthen bones and improve joint flexibility. Weight-bearing exercises stimulate bone growth and reduce the risk of osteoporosis and arthritis, promoting overall skeletal health.

6. Improved Sleep Quality: Jogging regulates sleep patterns, making it easier to fall asleep and stay asleep throughout the night. At age 40, prioritizing sleep becomes essential for overall health and well-being, and jogging can contribute to better sleep quality.

7. Sense of Achievement and Empowerment: Starting a jogging routine at 40 can instill a sense of accomplishment and empowerment. It's a tangible way to take control of your health and fitness, setting and achieving goals that boost confidence and self-esteem.

8. Longevity and Quality of Life: Regular jogging has been linked to increased longevity and improved quality of life. By promoting overall health and well-being, jogging at age 40 can help you enjoy a longer, healthier life with greater vitality and independence.

Overcoming Age-Related Obstacles

1. Starting Slow: Recognize that your body may not be as resilient as it once was, so it's important to start your jogging journey gradually. Begin with shorter distances and slower paces to allow your body to adapt and avoid overexertion.

2. Listening to Your Body: Pay attention to any signs of discomfort or pain during your jogging sessions. As you age, it's crucial to listen to your body and adjust your routine accordingly. Don't push through pain, as it could lead to injury.

3. Joint Health: Aging can sometimes bring about joint issues such as arthritis or stiffness. Choose appropriate footwear with good cushioning and support to minimize impact on your joints. Consider incorporating low-impact activities like swimming or cycling alongside jogging to reduce strain on your joints.

4. Muscle Strength and Flexibility: Aging often leads to a decline in muscle strength and flexibility. Incorporate regular strength training and stretching exercises into your routine to maintain muscle mass, improve flexibility, and prevent injuries.

5. Recovery Time: Allow for adequate rest and recovery between jogging sessions. As you get older, your body may take longer to recover from physical activity. Be mindful of this and prioritize rest days to prevent burnout and promote muscle repair.

6. Hydration and Nutrition: Aging can affect your body's ability to regulate temperature and hydration levels. Stay well-hydrated before, during, and after your runs, especially in hot weather. Additionally, focus on a balanced diet rich in nutrients to support your overall health and recovery.

7. Mindset Shift: Overcoming age-related obstacles also requires a shift in mindset. Embrace the journey and focus on progress rather than perfection. Celebrate small victories along the way and be patient with yourself as you work towards your jogging goals.

8. Seeking Professional Guidance: If you have any underlying health concerns or medical conditions, consult with a healthcare professional before starting a jogging routine. They can provide personalized advice and guidance to help you safely navigate any age-related obstacles.

By being mindful of these age-related obstacles and implementing appropriate strategies, you can overcome challenges and enjoy the many benefits that jogging has to offer well into your 40s and beyond. Remember, consistency and perseverance are key as you embark on this fulfilling journey towards improved health and well-being.

ASSESSING YOUR CURRENT FITNESS LEVEL

Before diving into a jogging routine at the age of 40, it's important to take stock of your current fitness level. This assessment serves as a baseline, helping you understand where you stand physically and what areas may need improvement.

Here are some key factors to consider:

Health Check-Up: Schedule a visit with your healthcare provider to assess your overall health and fitness readiness for jogging. Discuss any existing medical conditions, medications, or concerns that may impact your ability to engage in physical activity.

Physical Activity History: Reflect on your past experiences with exercise and physical activity. Have you been consistently active, or have there been periods of inactivity? Understanding your exercise history can provide insight into your fitness level and help set realistic goals.

Mobility and Flexibility: Evaluate your range of motion and flexibility in key joints and muscles. Are there any areas of stiffness or tightness that may affect your ability to jog comfortably? Incorporating stretching and mobility exercises can help improve flexibility and prevent injuries.

Cardiovascular Endurance: Assess your cardiovascular fitness by performing activities that elevate your heart rate, such as brisk walking or climbing stairs. Pay attention to how quickly you become winded and your ability to sustain activity over time.

Strength and Muscular Endurance: Gauge your muscular strength and endurance through bodyweight exercises like squats, lunges, and push-ups. Assess your ability to perform these movements with proper form and control, noting any areas of weakness or imbalance.

Balance and Coordination: Evaluate your balance and coordination, which are essential for safe and efficient movement while jogging. Practice simple balance exercises like standing on one leg or walking heel-to-toe to improve stability and control.

Mental Preparedness: Consider your mindset and motivation for starting a jogging routine. Are you mentally prepared to commit to regular exercise and overcome potential challenges along the way?

Cultivate a positive attitude and a growth mindset to stay focused and resilient throughout your fitness journey.

Health Check-Up

Prior to initiating a jogging regimen at the age of 40, it is prudent to undergo a comprehensive health assessment. This entails scheduling a consultation with a qualified healthcare professional, such as your primary care physician or a sports medicine specialist. During this examination, various aspects of your health and fitness will be evaluated to ensure that jogging is both safe and appropriate for you.

Key components of a health check-up may include:

Medical History: Your healthcare provider will review your medical history, including any pre-existing conditions, chronic illnesses, past surgeries, and current medications. This information helps assess your overall health status and identify any potential risk factors associated with jogging.

Physical Examination: A thorough physical examination will be conducted to assess your vital signs, cardiovascular health, respiratory function, musculoskeletal system, and overall fitness level. This may involve measuring your blood pressure, heart rate, lung function, and flexibility, as well as evaluating joint mobility and muscle strength.

Laboratory Tests: Depending on your individual health profile and risk factors, your healthcare provider may recommend certain laboratory tests to assess your baseline health parameters. These may include blood tests to measure cholesterol levels, blood sugar levels, and other markers of cardiovascular health, as well as tests to assess kidney and liver function.

Screening for Risk Factors: Your healthcare provider may inquire about lifestyle factors that could impact your ability to engage in physical activity safely, such as smoking, alcohol consumption, dietary habits, and stress levels. Additionally, they may screen for risk factors such as obesity, hypertension, diabetes, and family history of cardiovascular disease.

Exercise Tolerance: Your healthcare provider may assess your exercise tolerance through a graded exercise test or stress test, which involves monitoring your heart rate, blood pressure, and electrocardiogram (ECG) responses to physical exertion. This helps determine your cardiovascular fitness level and identify any underlying cardiac abnormalities that may warrant further evaluation.

Based on the findings of your health check-up, your healthcare provider will provide personalized recommendations regarding the safety and suitability of jogging for you. They may offer guidance on exercise intensity, duration, frequency, and any modifications needed to accommodate specific health concerns or limitations. Additionally, they can provide advice on injury prevention, proper warm-up and cool-down techniques, and strategies for monitoring your progress and adjusting your exercise regimen over time. Ultimately, undergoing a thorough health check-up before starting jogging at the age of 40 is essential for promoting optimal health, reducing the risk of injuries, and ensuring a positive and rewarding exercise experience.

Understanding Physical Limitations

Before embarking on a jogging routine at the age of 40, it's crucial to have a clear understanding of your physical limitations. As we age, our bodies undergo various changes that may affect our ability to engage in certain activities, including jogging.

 Here are some key considerations to keep in mind:

Assessing Joint Health: Take stock of any existing joint issues or conditions, such as arthritis or previous injuries that may impact your ability to jog comfortably. Listen to your body and pay attention to any discomfort or pain in your joints during and after jogging.

Muscle Strength and Flexibility: Be aware of any limitations in muscle strength and flexibility, which can affect your range of motion and overall mobility. Incorporate regular stretching and strength training exercises to improve flexibility and reduce the risk of muscle imbalances and injuries.

Cardiovascular Health: Consider any cardiovascular conditions or risk factors that may affect your ability to engage in aerobic exercise like jogging. If you have a history of heart disease, hypertension, or other cardiac issues, consult with your healthcare provider before starting a jogging routine.

Respiratory Function: Assess your respiratory function and lung capacity, particularly if you have a history of respiratory conditions such as asthma or chronic obstructive pulmonary disease (COPD). Monitor your breathing during exercise and seek medical advice if you experience difficulty breathing or chest tightness.

Balance and Coordination: Take note of any issues with balance and coordination, which can increase the risk of falls and injuries while jogging. Practice balance exercises and focus on maintaining proper form and stability during your runs.

Pacing Yourself: Recognize that your body may not recover as quickly as it did in your younger years. Start slowly and gradually increase the intensity and duration of your jogging sessions to avoid overexertion and minimize the risk of injury.

Listening to Your Body: Pay close attention to how your body responds to jogging and be prepared to modify your routine accordingly. If you experience persistent pain, fatigue, or other warning signs, take a break and consult with a healthcare professional if necessary.

Setting Realistic Goals

When starting a jogging routine at the age of 40, it's essential to set realistic and achievable goals that align with your current fitness level, lifestyle, and overall health. Setting realistic goals helps you stay motivated, track your progress, and maintain consistency in your jogging regimen.

Here are some key principles to keep in mind when setting goals:

Assess Your Starting Point: Before setting goals, take stock of your current fitness level and jogging ability. Consider factors such as your endurance, speed, and comfort level with running. This assessment will help you establish a baseline from which to set realistic goals.

Consider Your Health and Lifestyle: Take into account any health conditions, time constraints, or other commitments that may impact your jogging routine. Set goals that are compatible with your lifestyle and that prioritize your overall health and well-being.

Focus on Process Goals: Instead of solely focusing on outcome-based goals like weight loss or race times, prioritize process goals that emphasize consistent effort and improvement. For example, aim to jog a certain distance or duration each week, gradually increasing your mileage over time.

Be Specific and Measurable: Set clear and measurable goals that allow you to track your progress objectively. Instead of vague goals like "get in shape," set specific targets such as jogging three times per week or completing a 5,000 steps race within a certain timeframe.

Start Small and Build Gradually: Begin with attainable goals that are within your current capabilities, then gradually increase the intensity, duration, or frequency of your jogging sessions as you progress. This incremental approach helps prevent burnout and reduces the risk of injury.

Stay Flexible and Adapt: Be prepared to adjust your goals as needed based on your progress, changing circumstances, and feedback from your body. If you encounter setbacks or obstacles along the way, don't be discouraged—simply reassess your goals and make adjustments as necessary.

Celebrate Milestones: Acknowledge and celebrate your achievements along the way, no matter how small they may seem. Whether it's completing your first mile without stopping or achieving a new personal best, take pride in your progress and use it as motivation to keep pushing forward.

Setting realistic and achievable goals for your jogging routine at the age of 40, can make you establish a solid foundation for success and longevity in your fitness journey. Remember to prioritize consistency, patience, and self-care as you work towards your goals, and don't hesitate to seek support from friends, family, or fitness professionals if needed.

GETTING THE RIGHT GEAR

Ensuring you have the appropriate gear is essential for a comfortable and safe jogging experience, especially as you embark on this journey at the age of 40.

Here's what to consider when selecting your jogging gear:

Footwear: Invest in a good pair of running shoes that provide adequate cushioning, support, and stability. Look for shoes designed specifically for running and consider factors such as your foot type, gait, and any pronation issues. Get fitted by a knowledgeable salesperson at a specialty running store to find the right fit for your feet.

Clothing: Choose moisture-wicking and breathable fabrics that help keep you dry and comfortable during your runs. Opt for lightweight, loose-fitting clothing that allows for freedom of movement and prevents chafing. Consider wearing layers to accommodate changes in temperature and weather conditions.

Socks: Invest in high-quality running socks made from moisture-wicking materials to keep your feet dry and reduce the risk of blisters. Look for socks with cushioning in key areas such as the heel and forefoot to provide added comfort and protection.

Accessories: Consider any additional accessories that may enhance your jogging experience, such as a supportive sports bra for women, a hydration belt or water bottle for staying hydrated during longer runs, a GPS watch or smartphone app for tracking your distance and pace, and reflective gear or a headlamp for running in low-light conditions.

Safety Gear: Prioritize safety by wearing bright, reflective clothing and accessories to increase your visibility to motorists and other pedestrians, especially when running in dimly lit areas or during early morning or evening hours. Carry a form of identification and a cell phone with you in case of emergencies.

Sun Protection: Protect your skin from the sun's harmful rays by wearing sunscreen with a high SPF rating, sunglasses with UV protection, and a hat or visor to shield your face from direct sunlight.

Proper Hydration: Stay hydrated before, during, and after your runs by drinking water or a sports drink to replenish fluids lost through sweat. Consider carrying a handheld water bottle or wearing a hydration pack for longer runs.

Investing in the right gear tailored to your needs and preferences, you can enhance your comfort, safety, and enjoyment while jogging at the age of 40. Remember to replace worn-out shoes and clothing regularly to maintain optimal performance and minimize the risk of injury.

Choosing the Right Shoes

Selecting the appropriate footwear is perhaps the most critical aspect of gearing up for jogging at the age of 40. The right pair of shoes can make a significant difference in your comfort, performance, and injury prevention.

Here's what to consider when choosing running shoes:

Foot Type: Understand your foot type and biomechanics, including factors such as arch height, pronation (the inward rolling of the foot), and supination (the outward rolling of the foot). These factors can influence the type of shoe that best suits your needs.

Shoe Category: Running shoes come in various categories, including neutral, stability, and motion control, each designed to address different foot mechanics and provide varying levels of support and cushioning. Determine which category is most suitable for your foot type and running style.

Fit: Ensure proper fit by trying on shoes in the afternoon or evening when your feet are at their largest. Allow a thumb's width of space between your longest toe (usually the big toe) and the end of the shoe. Check for adequate width and volume to accommodate the natural swelling of your feet during exercise.

Comfort: Prioritize comfort above all else. Look for shoes with ample cushioning in the midsole to absorb impact and provide shock absorption. Pay attention to how the shoes feel on your feet, particularly in areas prone to rubbing or discomfort.

Flexibility: Test the flexibility of the shoes by bending them at the forefoot and heel. They should bend easily at the ball of the foot but offer some resistance at the arch and heel to provide stability and support.

Breathability: Choose shoes made from breathable materials that allow air to circulate and moisture to escape, helping keep your feet cool and dry during your runs. Look for mesh uppers and ventilation ports to enhance breathability.

Durability: Invest in high-quality shoes with durable construction and materials that can withstand the rigors of regular jogging. Check for reinforced areas such as the toe box and heel counter to ensure long-lasting wear.

Special Considerations: If you have specific foot issues or conditions such as plantar fasciitis, bunions, or over pronation, consult with a podiatrist or footwear specialist for personalized recommendations. They can help you select shoes with features tailored to address your unique needs and reduce the risk of discomfort or injury.

Ultimately, choosing the right shoes is a highly individualized process that depends on factors such as foot type, running mechanics, and personal preferences. Take the time to find the perfect pair that offers the support, comfort, and performance you need to enjoy jogging at the age of 40 to the fullest.

Comfortable Clothing for Jogging

When it comes to jogging at the age of 40, wearing comfortable clothing can make all the difference in your performance and enjoyment.

Here are some tips for selecting clothing that will keep you comfortable and motivated during your runs:

Fabric: Choose moisture-wicking fabrics such as polyester or nylon blends that help draw sweat away from your skin and allow it to evaporate quickly. These materials help keep you dry and comfortable, preventing chafing and irritation.

Fit: Opt for clothing that fits loosely and allows for freedom of movement. Avoid garments that are too tight or restrictive, as they can impede your stride and cause discomfort. Look for tops and bottoms with a relaxed fit that provide ample room to move.

Layering: Dress in layers to regulate your body temperature and adapt to changing weather conditions. Start with a moisture-wicking base layer to wick sweat away from your skin, add a lightweight mid-layer for insulation, and finish with a weather-resistant outer layer to protect against wind and rain.

Breathability: Choose clothing with breathable mesh panels or ventilation zones in areas prone to overheating, such as the underarms and back. These features help promote airflow and keep you cool and comfortable during your runs.

Sun Protection: Wear lightweight, long-sleeved tops and bottoms made from UPF-rated fabrics to protect your skin from the sun's harmful UV rays. Additionally, consider wearing a wide-brimmed hat or visor and sunglasses with UV protection to shield your face and eyes from sun exposure.

Visibility: Opt for bright, high-visibility clothing and accessories, especially if you'll be jogging in low-light conditions or during dawn or dusk. Choose garments with reflective elements or add reflective tape to your clothing and shoes to enhance your visibility to motorists and other pedestrians.

Seams and Construction: Look for clothing with flatlock seams and smooth, irritation-free construction to minimize chafing and rubbing. Avoid garments with bulky seams or rough edges that can cause discomfort during prolonged activity.

Accessorizing: Consider adding accessories such as moisture-wicking socks, sweat-wicking headbands or caps, and lightweight gloves or arm sleeves to enhance your comfort and performance during your runs.

Optional Accessories

While the essentials for jogging include proper footwear and comfortable clothing, there are several optional accessories that can enhance your experience and performance.

Consider incorporating these accessories into your jogging routine at the age of 40:

1. Running Watch or Fitness Tracker: A GPS-enabled running watch or fitness tracker can provide valuable data such as distance, pace, heart rate, and calories burned during your runs. This information allows you to track your progress, set goals, and monitor your performance over time.

2. Hydration Belt or Vest: Stay hydrated during longer runs by wearing a hydration belt or vest equipped with water bottles or a hydration bladder. These accessories allow you to carry water conveniently without disrupting your stride.

3. Running Belt or Waist Pack: A lightweight running belt or waist pack provides storage for essentials such as your phone, keys, ID, and energy gels or snacks. Choose a slim, low-profile design that won't bounce or chafe while jogging.

4. Reflective Gear: Enhance your visibility to motorists and other pedestrians by wearing reflective gear such as vests, armbands, or ankle bands. These accessories increase your safety when jogging in low-light conditions or at night.

5. Headlamp or Handheld Light: Illuminate your path and improve visibility during early morning or evening runs with a headlamp or handheld light. Choose a lightweight and adjustable light source that allows you to see and be seen while jogging in the dark.

6. Compression Socks or Sleeves: Improve circulation, reduce muscle fatigue, and enhance recovery by wearing compression socks or sleeves during and after your runs. These accessories provide targeted compression to key muscle groups and can help prevent injuries such as shin splints and calf cramps.

7. Foam Roller or Massage Ball: Incorporate self-massage and myofascial release into your post-run recovery routine with a foam roller or massage ball. These accessories help relieve muscle tension, improve flexibility, and accelerate recovery between workouts.

8. Sunglasses: Protect your eyes from glare, wind, and debris by wearing sunglasses with UV protection during your runs. Look for lightweight, wraparound styles that provide full coverage and a secure fit.

9. Hat or Visor: Shield your face and eyes from the sun's rays and keep sweat out of your eyes with a lightweight hat or visor. Choose a breathable and moisture-wicking material that helps keep you cool and comfortable during your runs.

10. Running Gloves: Keep your hands warm and comfortable during chilly weather runs with lightweight running gloves. Look for gloves made from moisture-wicking materials that provide warmth without bulkiness.

Incorporating these optional accessories into your jogging routine, you can enhance your comfort, safety, and performance while enjoying the many benefits of running at the age of 40. Experiment with different accessories to find the combination that works best for you and enhances your overall running experience.

Creating a Jogging Plan

As you embark on your jogging journey at the age of 40, it's essential to establish a structured plan that guides your training and progression. A well-designed jogging plan takes into account your current fitness level, goals, schedule, and any potential limitations or considerations.

Here's how to create a personalized jogging plan:

Assess Your Starting Point: Begin by assessing your current fitness level and jogging ability. Consider factors such as your endurance, speed, and comfort level with running. This assessment provides a baseline from which to tailor your jogging plan.

Set Realistic Goals: Define clear and achievable goals that align with your fitness aspirations. Whether you aim to improve cardiovascular health, increase endurance, or train for a specific event, set SMART goals that are Specific, Measurable, Attainable, Relevant, and Time-bound.

Determine Frequency: Decide how often you'll jog each week based on your schedule and fitness goals. Aim for consistency by scheduling regular sessions, but be flexible and allow for rest days to prevent burnout and promote recovery.

Plan Your Workouts: Structure your jogging plan with a mix of different types of workouts, including steady-state runs, interval training, and long runs. Varying your workouts helps prevent boredom, promotes fitness gains, and reduces the risk of overuse injuries.

Progress Gradually: Gradually increase the intensity, duration, and frequency of your jogging sessions over time to avoid overexertion and minimize the risk of injury. Follow the principle of progressive overload by challenging your body with incremental increases in workload.

Include Cross-Training: Incorporate cross-training activities such as cycling, swimming, or strength training into your jogging plan to improve overall fitness, prevent muscle imbalances, and reduce the risk of overuse injuries.

Warm-Up and Cool-Down: Prioritize warm-up and cool-down routines before and after your jogging sessions to prepare your body for exercise and promote recovery. Incorporate dynamic stretches, mobility exercises, and foam rolling to enhance flexibility and reduce muscle stiffness.

Listen to Your Body: Pay attention to how your body responds to training and be prepared to adjust your plan accordingly. If you experience persistent fatigue, soreness, or discomfort, consider taking a break or modifying your workouts to allow for adequate recovery.

Monitor Your Progress: Keep track of your workouts, progress, and achievements to stay motivated and accountable. Use a training log, fitness app, or wearable device to record data such as distance, pace, and heart rate.

Seek Support: Consider seeking guidance from a certified running coach, personal trainer, or experienced runner to help you design and implement an effective jogging plan. They can provide personalized advice, support, and motivation to help you reach your goals.

Determining Distance and Time

When planning your jogging sessions at the age of 40, it's important to consider both the distance and time you'll be covering to ensure that your workouts are effective and aligned with your fitness goals.

Distance: Decide on the distance you want to cover during each jogging session based on your current fitness level, goals, and available time. Start with shorter distances if you're new to jogging or gradually increase the distance as you build endurance and confidence. Consider factors such as terrain, elevation, and weather conditions when determining your route and distance.

Time: Determine the duration of your jogging sessions by setting a target amount of time to spend running. This approach allows for flexibility in your workouts and allows you to focus on effort rather than distance. Start with shorter time intervals, such as 20-30 minutes, and gradually increase the duration as your fitness improves. Listen to your body and adjust the intensity and duration of your runs as needed to avoid overexertion and fatigue.

Combining Distance and Time: Alternatively, you can set specific goals for both distance and time to structure your jogging sessions. For example, you might aim to jog a certain distance within a set time frame, such as completing a 5K (3.1 miles) in under 30 minutes.

This approach provides a clear target to work towards and allows you to track your progress over time.

Use Technology: Take advantage of technology such as GPS-enabled running watches or smartphone apps to track your distance, time, and pace during your jogging sessions. These tools provide valuable data that can help you monitor your progress, set goals, and stay motivated. Experiment with different apps and devices to find the one that best suits your needs and preferences.

Listen to Your Body: Regardless of the distance or time you choose for your jogging sessions, it's important to listen to your body and adjust your workouts accordingly. Pay attention to signs of fatigue, discomfort, or pain, and be prepared to modify your pace, duration, or route as needed. Remember that rest and recovery are just as important as training, so prioritize rest days and recovery activities to prevent burnout and promote overall well-being.

Incorporating Rest Days

Rest days are essential for optimizing recovery, preventing overuse injuries, and promoting overall well-being, especially when incorporating jogging into your routine at the age of 40. Here are some key considerations for incorporating rest days into your jogging schedule:

Frequency: Schedule rest days into your jogging plan at regular intervals to allow your body time to recover and repair between workouts. Aim for at least one or two rest days per week, depending on your fitness level, training intensity, and individual recovery needs.

Strategic Placement: Strategically place rest days after harder or more challenging workouts to facilitate recovery and adaptation. For example, schedule a rest day following a long run, interval training session, or race to allow your muscles time to recover and rebuild.

Active Recovery: Consider incorporating active recovery activities on rest days to promote circulation, flexibility, and muscle relaxation. Light activities such as walking, cycling, swimming, or yoga can help facilitate recovery without placing additional stress on your muscles and joints.

Listen to Your Body: Pay attention to how your body feels and adjust your rest days accordingly. If you experience persistent fatigue, soreness, or signs of overtraining, consider taking an extra rest day or reducing the intensity of your workouts. Remember that rest days are not a sign of weakness but rather an essential component of a balanced training regimen.

Mental Rest: In addition to physical rest, prioritize mental rest and relaxation on rest days. Use this time to recharge, de-stress, and engage in activities that promote mental well-being, such as meditation, mindfulness, or spending time with loved ones.

Flexibility: Be flexible with your rest day schedule and adapt as needed based on your energy levels, recovery status, and other commitments. It's okay to shift rest days around or take an unplanned rest day if life gets busy or your body needs extra recovery time.

Long-Term Planning: Incorporate rest days into your long-term training plan to prevent burnout and sustain your motivation and enthusiasm for jogging over time. Remember that consistency and sustainability are key to long-term success in fitness and health.

By incorporating rest days into your jogging routine at the age of 40, you can optimize your recovery, reduce the risk of injury, and maintain a healthy balance between training and rest. Prioritize rest, listen to your body, and enjoy the benefits of a well-rounded approach to fitness and well-being.

STARTING SLOW: BUILDING ENDURANCE SAFELY

When beginning a jogging routine at the age of 40, it's crucial to start slow and gradually build endurance to reduce the risk of injury and ensure long-term success. This gradual approach allows your body to adapt to the demands of jogging while minimizing the likelihood of overexertion or burnout.

Begin by setting realistic expectations and accepting that progress may take time. Start with shorter distances and slower paces than you may initially desire, focusing on establishing a consistent routine rather than pushing yourself too hard too soon.

Listen to your body and pay attention to how it responds to jogging. Start with a comfortable pace that allows you to maintain a conversation without feeling out of breath. As you become more comfortable with jogging, gradually increase the duration and intensity of your runs.

Incorporate walk breaks as needed to manage fatigue and maintain a sustainable effort level. Start with a run-walk approach, alternating periods of jogging with brief walking intervals to allow for active recovery. As your endurance improves, gradually reduce the duration of walk breaks and increase the duration of continuous running segments.

Be patient and allow yourself time to progress at your own pace. It's normal to experience setbacks or plateaus along the way, but consistency and perseverance are key to building endurance safely. Celebrate small victories and milestones as you progress, whether it's completing your first mile without stopping or increasing your overall distance.

Gradually increase the volume and intensity of your jogging workouts over time, but be mindful of the 10% rule—avoid increasing your weekly mileage or intensity by more than 10% from one week to the next to prevent overuse injuries.

Incorporate cross-training activities such as cycling, swimming, or strength training to complement your jogging routine and improve overall fitness. Cross-training helps prevent overuse injuries, promotes muscle balance, and enhances cardiovascular health.

Prioritize rest and recovery to allow your body time to adapt and repair between workouts. Adequate sleep, proper nutrition, hydration, and stress management are essential components of a well-rounded training regimen.

Remember that building endurance is a gradual process that requires patience, consistency, and dedication. By starting slow and progressing steadily, you can safely increase your endurance and enjoy the many benefits of jogging at the age of 40 for years to come.

Warm-Up and Cool-Down Routines

Incorporating warm-up and cool-down routines into your jogging regimen at the age of 40 is essential for preparing your body for exercise, preventing injuries, and promoting recovery. Here's how to structure effective warm-up and cool-down routines:

Warm-Up:

- Begin your warm-up with 5-10 minutes of low-intensity cardiovascular activity, such as brisk walking, light jogging, or cycling. This helps increase blood flow to your muscles and prepares your body for more intense exercise.

- Incorporate dynamic stretches and mobility exercises to loosen up your muscles and joints. Focus on movements that mimic the actions you'll be performing during your jog, such as leg swings, arm circles, hip circles, and lunges.

- Gradually increase the intensity of your warm-up by incorporating short bursts of higher-intensity activity, such as skipping, high knees, or butt kicks. This helps elevate your heart rate and primes your muscles for the demands of jogging.

Cool-Down:

- After completing your jogging session, gradually reduce the intensity of your activity by transitioning to a slower pace or walking. This helps lower your heart rate and prevent blood from pooling in your lower extremities.

- Perform static stretches targeting the major muscle groups used during jogging, holding each stretch for 15-30 seconds without bouncing. Focus on areas such as your calves, quadriceps, hamstrings, hips, and lower back. Remember to stretch both sides of your body evenly.

- Incorporate foam rolling or self-massage techniques to release tension and promote muscle relaxation. Use a foam roller or massage ball to target areas of tightness and trigger points, applying gentle pressure and rolling back and forth over the affected muscles.

- Hydrate and refuel your body with water and a nutritious post-workout snack or meal to replenish glycogen stores and support muscle recovery. Aim to consume a combination of carbohydrates and protein within 30-60 minutes of completing your jog to optimize recovery.

Incorporating warm-up and cool-down routines into your jogging regimen, you can enhance performance, reduce the risk of injuries, and promote overall well-being at the age of 40. Prioritize consistency and mindfulness in your warm-up and cool-down practices, and listen to your body to determine what works best for you.

Interval Training for Beginners

Interval training is a highly effective and efficient method for improving cardiovascular fitness, boosting metabolism, and burning calories, making it an excellent option for beginners starting a jogging regimen at the age of 40. Interval training alternates between periods of high-intensity exercise and periods of lower-intensity recovery or rest, allowing you to push your limits while still accommodating your current fitness level.

Here's how to incorporate interval training into your jogging routine as a beginner:

Begin by selecting a suitable location for your interval workout, such as a flat stretch of road or a track with marked distances. Alternatively, you can use a treadmill with adjustable speed settings for indoor workouts.

Start with a 5-10 minute warm-up of light jogging or brisk walking to prepare your body for the workout ahead. Focus on gradually increasing your heart rate and loosening up your muscles and joints.

Once you're warmed up, begin your first interval by jogging at a moderate to high intensity for a predetermined period of time, such as 30 seconds to 1 minute. Aim to push yourself to a challenging pace that elevates your heart rate and leaves you feeling breathless but still able to maintain good form.

After completing the high-intensity interval, transition into a recovery period of low-intensity jogging or walking for an equal or slightly longer duration than the interval itself. Use this recovery period to catch your breath, lower your heart rate, and prepare for the next interval.

Repeat this cycle of high-intensity intervals followed by recovery periods for a total of 5-10 intervals, depending on your fitness level and tolerance. Gradually increase the duration or intensity of your intervals as you become more comfortable with the workout.

Finish your interval training session with a 5-10 minute cool-down of light jogging or walking to gradually lower your heart rate and promote recovery. Use this time to stretch your muscles and focus on deep breathing to help your body transition back to a resting state.

Interval training can be customized to suit your individual fitness goals and preferences. Experiment with different interval lengths, intensities, and recovery durations to find the combination that works best for you. Remember to listen to your body and adjust the workout as needed to ensure safety and enjoyment.

Incorporate interval training into your jogging routine 1-2 times per week, alternating with steady-state runs or other forms of cardiovascular exercise to maintain a balanced training regimen. With consistent practice and gradual progression, interval training can help you build endurance, increase speed, and achieve your fitness goals at the age of 40 and beyond.

Gradual Progression Techniques

Gradual progression is the cornerstone of any successful fitness regimen, especially when starting a jogging routine at the age of 40. By gradually increasing the intensity, duration, and frequency of your workouts over time, you can build endurance, improve fitness, and minimize the risk of injury.

Here are some gradual progression techniques to incorporate into your jogging routine:

1. Start Slow: Begin your jogging journey at a comfortable pace that allows you to maintain good form and breathe easily. Start with shorter distances and slower speeds than you may initially desire, focusing on establishing a consistent routine rather than pushing yourself too hard too soon.

2. Incremental Increases: Gradually increase the intensity, duration, and frequency of your jogging workouts in small, manageable increments. For example, add an extra minute or two to your run each week, or increase your weekly mileage by no more than 10% to prevent overuse injuries.

3. Listen to Your Body: Pay attention to how your body responds to jogging and adjust your workouts accordingly. If you experience persistent fatigue, soreness, or signs of overtraining, consider taking a step back and reducing the intensity or duration of your runs.

4. Mix It Up: Incorporate variety into your jogging routine by mixing up your workouts with different types of runs, such as steady-state runs, interval training, and long runs. Varying your workouts helps prevent boredom, promotes fitness gains, and reduces the risk of overuse injuries.

5. Rest and Recovery: Prioritize rest and recovery to allow your body time to adapt and repair between workouts. Incorporate rest days into your training schedule, and listen to your body's cues for when to take additional rest or recovery days as needed.

6. Set Realistic Goals: Set clear and achievable goals that align with your current fitness level and aspirations. Break larger goals into smaller, more manageable milestones, and celebrate your progress along the way.

7. Track Your Progress: Keep a training log or use a fitness app to track your workouts, progress, and achievements. Monitoring your performance allows you to see how far you've come and helps keep you motivated and accountable.

8. Be Patient and Consistent: Rome wasn't built in a day, and neither is endurance or fitness. Be patient with yourself and trust the process of gradual progression. Stay consistent with your workouts, even on days when motivation is low, and remember that every step forward, no matter how small, is a step in the right direction.

PROPER RUNNING TECHNIQUE

Maintaining proper running technique is essential for maximizing efficiency, preventing injuries, and enhancing performance, especially as you embark on jogging at the age of 40.

Here are some key elements of proper running technique to keep in mind:

1. Posture: Maintain an upright posture with your head facing forward and your shoulders relaxed and down. Keep your spine straight and avoid slouching or leaning forward at the waist. Engage your core muscles to stabilize your torso and maintain balance as you run.

2. Arm Movement: Swing your arms naturally in a relaxed and controlled manner, allowing them to move in coordination with your leg stride. Keep your elbows bent at approximately 90 degrees and your hands relaxed, with your arms swinging back and forth along your sides rather than crossing over your body.

3. Cadence: Aim for a quick and efficient cadence of around 170-180 steps per minute, regardless of your running speed. Focus on shortening your stride and increasing your turnover rate rather than

taking long, bounding strides. A higher cadence helps reduce impact forces, improve efficiency, and reduce the risk of injury.

4. Foot Strike: Land softly and quietly on your midfoot or forefoot with each step, rather than striking the ground with your heel first. Aim to land with your foot directly underneath your body, minimizing over striding and excessive braking forces. Focus on a smooth and fluid transition from landing to toe-off with each stride.

5. Knee Lift: Lift your knees slightly with each stride, aiming for a relaxed and natural movement that allows for efficient forward propulsion. Avoid excessive knee lift or exaggerated leg movements, as this can lead to wasted energy and increased fatigue.

6. Breathing: Focus on relaxed and rhythmic breathing to supply oxygen to your muscles and regulate your effort level. Breathe deeply from your diaphragm, inhaling through your nose and exhaling through your mouth. Find a breathing pattern that feels comfortable and sustainable for the duration of your run.

7. Relaxation: Stay relaxed and loose throughout your body, avoiding tension or stiffness in your muscles and joints. Relax your hands, arms, shoulders, and facial muscles, allowing for a smooth and efficient running motion. Pay attention to areas of tension or tightness and consciously release any areas of holding or stiffness.

8. Mindfulness: Stay present and mindful during your runs, paying attention to how your body feels and making adjustments as needed. Listen to your body's cues for signs of fatigue, discomfort, or imbalances, and make modifications to your technique or pace accordingly.

Focusing on these key elements of proper running technique and practicing mindfulness and awareness during your runs, can improve your efficiency, reduce the risk of injury, and enjoy a more enjoyable and fulfilling jogging experience at the age of 40 and beyond.

Posture and Form

Maintaining proper posture and form is crucial for optimizing performance, preventing injuries, and ensuring a enjoyable jogging experience, particularly as you start jogging at the age of 40. Here's how to focus on posture and form during your runs:

Posture:

Maintain an upright posture with your head facing forward and your gaze focused ahead. Avoid slouching or leaning forward at the waist, as this can strain your lower back and impair your breathing.

Keep your shoulders relaxed and down, away from your ears. Avoid tensing your shoulders or hunching them forward, as this can lead to tension and discomfort.

Engage your core muscles to stabilize your torso and maintain proper alignment. Imagine drawing your navel toward your spine to activate your abdominal muscles and support your posture.

Form:

Focus on a midfoot or forefoot strike rather than landing heavily on your heels. Aim to land softly and quietly with each step, using your foot's natural shock absorption to cushion the impact.

Keep your arms relaxed and swinging naturally in rhythm with your stride. Bend your elbows at approximately 90 degrees and avoid crossing your arms in front of your body.

Maintain a quick and efficient cadence of around 170-180 steps per minute. Focus on shortening your stride and increasing your turnover rate to reduce ground contact time and minimize impact forces.

Drive your arms back and forth in a controlled manner, keeping them close to your body. Avoid excessive arm movement or swinging your arms across your body, as this can waste energy and throw off your balance.

Focus on a smooth and fluid running motion, allowing your body to move naturally and efficiently. Avoid tensing up or forcing your movements, and instead strive for a relaxed and flowing stride.

In paying attention to your posture and form during your runs, you can improve efficiency, reduce the risk of injury, and enhance your overall running experience. Incorporate these tips into your jogging routine to maximize your performance and enjoyment at the age of 40 and beyond.

Breathing Techniques

Proper breathing techniques are essential for optimizing oxygen intake, maintaining endurance, and enhancing performance during jogging, especially as you start at the age of 40.

Here are some tips to help you develop effective breathing habits:

1. Breathe Deeply: Focus on breathing deeply from your diaphragm to maximize oxygen exchange and support your running effort. Inhale deeply through your nose, allowing your abdomen to expand, and exhale fully through your mouth, releasing tension and waste gases from your body.

2. Establish a Rhythm: Find a breathing rhythm that feels comfortable and sustainable for the duration of your run. Aim for a consistent breathing pattern, such as inhaling for two steps and exhaling for two steps, or inhaling for three steps and exhaling for two steps. Experiment with different patterns to find what works best for you.

3. Coordinate with Your Stride: Coordinate your breathing with your stride to maintain a smooth and efficient running motion. Try to time your inhales and exhales with your foot strikes, syncing your breathing with your natural cadence and rhythm.

4. Focus on Relaxation: Stay relaxed and loose as you breathe, avoiding tension or tightness in your chest, shoulders, or neck. Relax your facial muscles, jaw, and throat, allowing for easy and unrestricted airflow. Consciously release any areas of tension or holding in your body as you breathe.

5. Practice Belly Breathing: Practice belly breathing to engage your diaphragm and optimize oxygen intake. Place one hand on your chest and the other on your abdomen, and focus on breathing deeply into your belly rather than shallowly into your chest. Feel your abdomen rise and fall with each breath as you engage your diaphragm.

6. Be Mindful: Stay present and mindful of your breathing during your runs, using it as a focal point to anchor your attention and maintain focus. Pay attention to the rhythm, depth, and quality of your breath, and make adjustments as needed to ensure smooth and efficient breathing.

7. Relaxation Techniques: Incorporate relaxation techniques such as deep breathing exercises, visualization, or mindfulness meditation into your pre-run routine to help calm your mind and prepare your body for exercise. Use these techniques to reduce stress, anxiety, or tension that may interfere with your breathing during your run.

Avoiding Common Injuries

Preventing injuries is crucial for maintaining a consistent jogging routine and enjoying long-term health and fitness benefits, especially as you start at the age of 40.

Here are some strategies to help you avoid common injuries while jogging:

1. Gradual Progression: Gradually increase the intensity, duration, and frequency of your jogging workouts over time to allow your body to adapt and build strength. Avoid sudden spikes in training volume or intensity, as this can increase the risk of overuse injuries.

2. Proper Warm-Up and Cool-Down: Always start your jogging sessions with a thorough warm-up to prepare your muscles, joints, and cardiovascular system for exercise. Incorporate dynamic stretches, mobility exercises, and light cardio to increase blood flow and flexibility. Similarly, cool down with gentle jogging or walking and static stretching to promote recovery and reduce muscle stiffness.

3. Listen to Your Body: Pay attention to warning signs such as persistent pain, discomfort, or unusual sensations during or after your runs. If you experience pain that doesn't improve with rest, seek professional medical advice to identify and address any underlying issues.

4. Wear Appropriate Footwear: Invest in a pair of high-quality running shoes that provide adequate support, cushioning, and stability for your feet and gait. Replace your shoes regularly, typically every 300-500 miles or when signs of wear and tear appear, to ensure optimal protection and performance.

5. Cross-Train: Incorporate cross-training activities such as swimming, cycling, yoga, or strength training into your fitness routine to reduce the risk of overuse injuries and promote overall muscular balance and flexibility. Varying your workouts helps prevent repetitive strain on specific muscles and joints.

6. Strengthening Exercises: Include strength training exercises targeting key muscle groups such as the core, hips, glutes, and legs to improve stability, balance, and resilience. Focus on exercises that mimic running movements, such as squats, lunges, calf raises, and planks, to enhance muscular endurance and reduce the risk of imbalances and injuries.

7. Flexibility and Mobility: Incorporate regular stretching, foam rolling, and mobility exercises into your routine to improve flexibility, reduce muscle tension, and enhance joint range of motion. Focus on areas prone to tightness or stiffness, such as the calves, hamstrings, quadriceps, hips, and lower back.

8. Hydration and Nutrition: Stay hydrated and fuel your body with a balanced diet rich in nutrients, vitamins, and minerals to support overall health and recovery. Drink plenty of water before, during, and after your runs, and consume a combination of carbohydrates, protein, and healthy fats to replenish energy stores and support muscle repair and growth.

NUTRITION AND HYDRATION

Proper nutrition and hydration are essential components of a successful jogging routine, especially as you begin at the age of 40. Here's how to fuel your body for optimal performance and recovery:

Nutrition:

Focus on a balanced diet that includes a variety of nutrient-dense foods to support your overall health and fitness goals. Aim to include a combination of carbohydrates, protein, healthy fats, vitamins, and minerals in your meals and snacks.

Prioritize carbohydrates as the main source of energy for your runs, as they provide readily available fuel for your muscles. Include complex carbohydrates such as whole grains, fruits, vegetables, and legumes in your diet to provide sustained energy and support glycogen stores.

Consume an adequate amount of protein to support muscle repair and growth, especially after intense workouts or strength training sessions. Include lean sources of protein such as poultry, fish, eggs, tofu, legumes, and dairy products in your meals and snacks.

Incorporate healthy fats into your diet to support overall health and provide long-lasting energy. Include sources of unsaturated fats such as nuts, seeds, avocados, olive oil, and fatty fish in moderation.

Stay hydrated throughout the day by drinking water regularly and paying attention to your thirst cues. Aim to drink at least 8-10 cups of water per day, or more if you're exercising intensely or in hot weather.

Hydration:

Hydrate before, during, and after your runs to maintain fluid balance and prevent dehydration. Drink water or a sports drink containing electrolytes before your run to ensure adequate hydration and electrolyte levels.

During your runs, sip water or a sports drink at regular intervals to replenish fluids and electrolytes lost through sweat. Adjust your fluid intake based on the duration and intensity of your run, as well as environmental conditions such as temperature and humidity.

After your runs, rehydrate with water or a recovery drink containing electrolytes to replenish fluid and electrolyte losses and support muscle recovery. Aim to drink enough fluids to replace any weight lost during your run and hydrate your body for optimal recovery.

Listen to your body's thirst signals and adjust your fluid intake accordingly. Pay attention to signs of dehydration such as dark urine, dry mouth, dizziness, or fatigue, and drink fluids promptly to rehydrate.

By prioritizing proper nutrition and hydration, you can fuel your body for success and support your jogging routine at the age of 40 and beyond. Focus on consuming a balanced diet rich in carbohydrates, protein, and healthy fats, and stay hydrated by drinking water regularly before, during, and after your runs. With the right fuel and hydration strategy, you can optimize your performance, recovery, and overall well-being.

Pre-Run Fueling

Before heading out for a jog, it's important to fuel your body with the right nutrients to provide energy and support optimal performance. Here are some pre-run fueling strategies to consider:

1. Timing: Aim to eat a balanced meal or snack containing carbohydrates, protein, and a small amount of healthy fats 1-2 hours before your run. This allows time for digestion and absorption of nutrients, providing you with sustained energy without feeling overly full or sluggish.

2. Carbohydrates: Prioritize carbohydrates as the main source of energy for your pre-run meal or snack. Choose complex carbohydrates such as whole grains, fruits, vegetables, and legumes, which provide a steady release of glucose into the bloodstream to fuel your muscles during exercise.

3. Protein: Include a moderate amount of protein in your pre-run meal or snack to support muscle repair and growth. Choose lean sources of protein such as poultry, fish, eggs, tofu, yogurt, or nuts, which are easily digestible and provide essential amino acids for muscle recovery.

4. Hydration: Drink water or a sports drink containing electrolytes in the hours leading up to your run to ensure adequate hydration. Aim to drink enough fluids to maintain urine color that is pale yellow or straw-colored, indicating proper hydration status.

5. Avoid High-Fat or High-Fiber Foods: Avoid consuming high-fat or high-fiber foods immediately before your run, as they can slow digestion and cause gastrointestinal discomfort. Opt for lighter, easily digestible options that won't weigh you down or cause digestive issues during your run.

6. Experiment and Listen to Your Body: Experiment with different pre-run meals and snacks to find what works best for you. Pay attention to how different foods make you feel during your runs and

adjust your pre-run fueling strategy accordingly. Some runners may prefer a small snack, such as a banana with nut butter or a yogurt parfait, while others may prefer a larger meal, such as oatmeal with fruit and yogurt.

7. Avoid Overeating: Avoid consuming large or heavy meals immediately before your run, as they can lead to gastrointestinal distress and discomfort. Instead, opt for smaller, lighter meals or snacks that provide adequate energy without causing digestive issues.

Hydration Strategies

Proper hydration is essential for maintaining performance, preventing dehydration, and supporting overall health during jogging. Here are some hydration strategies to consider:

- Drink water regularly throughout the day to maintain hydration levels. Aim to drink at least 8-10 cups of water per day, or more if you're exercising intensely or in hot weather.

- Hydrate before your run by drinking water or a sports drink containing electrolytes in the hours leading up to your workout. Aim to drink 16-20 ounces of fluid 2-3 hours before your run to ensure adequate hydration.

- During your run, sip water or a sports drink at regular intervals to replenish fluids and electrolytes lost through sweat. Adjust your fluid intake based on the duration and intensity of your run, as well as environmental conditions such as temperature and humidity.

- Pay attention to your thirst cues and drink fluids promptly when you feel thirsty. Thirst is a sign that your body needs hydration, so listen to your body and respond accordingly.

- Consider using a hydration belt, handheld water bottle, or hydration pack to carry fluids with you during your run, especially for longer distances or in hot weather. Experiment with different hydration options to find what works best for you.

- Monitor your urine color to gauge hydration status. Aim for pale yellow or straw-colored urine, which indicates proper hydration. Dark urine may be a sign of dehydration and should prompt you to drink more fluids.

- Rehydrate after your run by drinking water or a recovery drink containing electrolytes to replenish fluid and electrolyte losses and support muscle recovery. Aim to drink enough fluids to replace any weight lost during your run and hydrate your body for optimal recovery.

Post-Run Recovery Meals

After completing a jog, it's important to refuel your body with the nutrients it needs to support muscle recovery, replenish energy stores, and promote overall recovery. Here are some post-run recovery meal ideas to consider:

1. Protein-Rich Smoothie: Blend together Greek yogurt, banana, spinach, protein powder, and almond milk for a delicious and nutrient-packed post-run smoothie. The combination of protein and carbohydrates helps repair muscles and replenish glycogen stores, while the fruits and vegetables provide essential vitamins and minerals.

2. Quinoa Salad: Toss cooked quinoa with mixed greens, cherry tomatoes, cucumbers, avocado, grilled chicken or tofu, and a drizzle of olive oil and balsamic vinegar. Quinoa is a complete protein that provides all nine essential amino acids, while the vegetables add fiber, vitamins, and antioxidants to support recovery and overall health.

3. Whole Grain Toast with Nut Butter: Spread whole grain toast with almond butter or peanut butter and top with sliced banana or strawberries for a simple and satisfying post-run snack. The combination of carbohydrates and protein helps replenish energy stores and repair muscles, while the fruit adds natural sweetness and additional nutrients.

4. Salmon with Sweet Potatoes and Steamed Vegetables: Grill or bake a piece of salmon and serve it with roasted sweet potatoes and steamed broccoli or asparagus. Salmon is rich in omega-3 fatty acids, which have anti-inflammatory properties and support muscle recovery, while sweet potatoes provide complex carbohydrates and vitamins.

5. Greek Yogurt Parfait: Layer Greek yogurt with granola, mixed berries, and a drizzle of honey for a nutritious and delicious post-run treat. Greek yogurt is high in protein and probiotics, which support muscle repair and digestive health, while the berries add antioxidants and fiber.

6. Turkey and Veggie Wrap: Fill a whole grain wrap with sliced turkey breast, hummus, spinach, shredded carrots, and sliced bell peppers for a portable and protein-packed post-run meal. The combination of lean protein, carbohydrates, and vegetables provides essential nutrients for recovery and refueling.

7. Bean and Vegetable Chili: Prepare a hearty bean and vegetable chili with kidney beans, black beans, diced tomatoes, onions, bell peppers, and spices such as chili powder, cumin, and paprika. Serve with a side of whole grain bread or brown rice for a satisfying and nourishing post-run meal.

Choosing nutrient-dense foods that provide a balance of carbohydrates, protein, healthy fats, vitamins, and minerals, you can support muscle recovery, replenish energy stores, and promote overall well-being after a jog. Experiment with different post-run meals and snacks to find what works best for you, and prioritize nourishing your body to maximize recovery and performance.

LISTENING TO YOUR BODY

One of the most important aspects of starting a jogging routine at the age of 40 is learning to listen to your body and respond to its cues. Your body has a remarkable ability to communicate its needs, signals, and limitations, and tuning into these messages is essential for staying healthy, preventing injuries, and optimizing performance.

Here are some ways to listen to your body:

Pay attention to how you feel before, during, and after your runs. Notice any sensations of fatigue, discomfort, pain, or tightness, as well as feelings of energy, strength, and satisfaction. Your body is constantly sending you signals about its state of health and well-being, so take the time to tune in and acknowledge these messages.

Learn to differentiate between normal sensations of fatigue or muscle soreness and signs of potential injury or overtraining. While some degree of discomfort or fatigue is normal during exercise, persistent pain or discomfort that worsens with activity may indicate an underlying issue that requires attention. Trust your instincts and seek professional medical advice if you're unsure about any symptoms or concerns.

Be mindful of your breathing, heart rate, and energy levels during your runs. Notice any changes or fluctuations in your breathing pattern, heart rate, or perceived exertion, and adjust your pace or intensity accordingly. Pay attention to how different factors such as weather, terrain, and hydration levels affect your performance and comfort level.

Take note of your mental and emotional state during your runs. Notice any feelings of stress, anxiety, or distraction, as well as moments of calm, focus, and joy. Running can be a powerful tool for improving mental health and well-being, so be present in the moment and allow yourself to fully experience the benefits of your workouts.

Practice self-care and prioritize rest and recovery as needed. Listen to your body's signals for rest, relaxation, and recovery, and honor these needs by taking rest days, incorporating active recovery activities, and getting adequate sleep and nutrition. Remember that rest is an essential part of the training process and allows your body to adapt and recover from the demands of exercise.

Trust your body's wisdom and intuition, and don't be afraid to modify your workouts or make adjustments as needed. Your body knows what it needs to thrive, so listen to its guidance and honor its messages. By cultivating a deeper awareness and connection with your body, you can enhance your running experience, improve your health and fitness, and enjoy the many benefits of jogging at the age of 40 and beyond.

Recognizing Signs of Overexertion

Overexertion occurs when you push your body beyond its limits, leading to physical and mental strain that can compromise your health and performance. Recognizing the signs of overexertion is crucial for preventing injuries and promoting overall well-being, especially when starting a jogging routine at the age of 40.

Here are some common signs of overexertion to watch for:

1. Persistent Fatigue: Feeling excessively tired or fatigued, even after adequate rest and recovery, may indicate that you're overexerting yourself. Pay attention to feelings of extreme tiredness that persist for an extended period of time, as this may be a sign that you need to dial back your training intensity or volume.

2. Increased Resting Heart Rate: Monitoring your resting heart rate can provide valuable insights into your body's recovery status and overall stress level. If you notice a sustained increase in your resting

heart rate over time, it may be a sign that you're overtraining and need to give your body more time to rest and recover.

3. Persistent Muscle Soreness: It's normal to experience muscle soreness after a challenging workout, but persistent or excessive soreness that doesn't improve with rest may indicate that you're overexerting yourself. Listen to your body and give yourself adequate time to recover between workouts to prevent overuse injuries.

4. Decreased Performance: If you notice a sudden decline in your performance or difficulty maintaining your usual pace or intensity during workouts, it may be a sign of overexertion. Pay attention to changes in your running form, speed, or endurance, and consider taking a step back to reassess your training approach.

5. Mood Changes: Overexertion can take a toll on your mental and emotional well-being, leading to mood changes such as irritability, anxiety, or depression. If you notice negative changes in your mood or outlook, it may be a sign that you're pushing yourself too hard and need to prioritize self-care and recovery.

6. Increased Injury Risk: Overexertion can increase your risk of injuries such as muscle strains, stress fractures, and tendonitis. If you're experiencing frequent or recurring injuries, it may be a sign

that you're overtraining and need to adjust your training volume, intensity, or frequency to prevent further damage.

7. Insomnia or Disrupted Sleep Patterns: Overexertion can disrupt your sleep patterns and lead to insomnia or difficulty falling asleep or staying asleep. Pay attention to changes in your sleep quality or duration, as poor sleep can impair recovery and negatively impact your overall health and well-being.

Recognizing these signs of overexertion and responding accordingly, you can avoid burnout, prevent injuries, and promote long-term health and performance in your jogging routine at the age of 40 and beyond. Listen to your body's signals, prioritize rest and recovery, and adjust your training approach as needed to support your health and fitness goals.

Adjusting Your Plan Accordingly

Flexibility and adaptability are key components of a successful jogging routine, especially as you navigate the unique challenges and changes that may arise at the age of 40. Adjusting your plan accordingly allows you to respond to your body's needs, accommodate unexpected circumstances, and maintain consistency and progress in your fitness journey.

Here are some strategies for adjusting your plan as needed:

Listen to Your Body: Pay attention to your body's signals and respond accordingly. If you're experiencing signs of fatigue, overexertion, or injury, don't hesitate to scale back your training intensity, volume, or frequency. Listen to your body's need for rest and recovery, and prioritize self-care to support your overall health and well-being.

Be Flexible: Recognize that life is unpredictable, and be prepared to adjust your plan based on changing circumstances. Whether its unexpected work commitments, family responsibilities, or unforeseen events, be willing to adapt your schedule and workout routine as needed to maintain consistency and progress towards your goals.

Set Realistic Expectations: Be realistic about what you can realistically achieve given your current circumstances, fitness level, and lifestyle. Set achievable goals and be willing to adjust your expectations as needed to avoid frustration or disappointment. Remember that progress is not always linear, and setbacks are a natural part of the journey.

Embrace Variety: Incorporate variety into your training routine to prevent boredom, reduce the risk of overuse injuries, and keep your workouts fresh and enjoyable. Mix up your workouts with different types of runs, cross-training activities, and recovery modalities to challenge your body in new ways and support overall fitness and well-being.

Seek Support and Guidance: Don't hesitate to seek support and guidance from qualified professionals such as coaches, trainers, or healthcare providers. A knowledgeable coach or trainer can help you create a customized training plan, provide expert advice on technique and form, and offer encouragement and motivation to help you reach your goals.

Stay Positive and Patient: Stay positive and patient with yourself as you navigate the ups and downs of your fitness journey. Remember that progress takes time, and setbacks are opportunities for growth and learning. Stay focused on your long-term goals, and celebrate your achievements along the way, no matter how small.

By staying flexible, listening to your body, and adjusting your plan accordingly, you can maintain consistency, progress, and enjoyment in your jogging routine at the age of 40 and beyond. Embrace the journey, stay committed to your goals, and trust in your ability to adapt and thrive in the face of challenges.

Incorporating Cross-Training

Cross-training is a valuable addition to any jogging routine, providing numerous benefits such as improved fitness, reduced risk of injury, and enhanced overall performance.

Here are some strategies for incorporating cross-training into your jogging routine:

1. Choose Activities You Enjoy: Select cross-training activities that you genuinely enjoy and look forward to. Whether it's swimming, cycling, yoga, strength training, or hiking, find activities that complement your jogging routine and align with your interests and preferences.

2. Mix up Your Workouts: Vary your cross-training activities to challenge your body in different ways and prevent boredom. Rotate between different activities throughout the week, incorporating a mix of cardiovascular exercise, strength training, flexibility work, and balance exercises to promote overall fitness and well-being.

3. Cross-Train on Rest Days: Use rest days as an opportunity to engage in low-impact cross-training activities that promote recovery and enhance overall fitness. Consider activities such as gentle yoga, swimming, or walking to keep your body moving while giving your muscles a chance to rest and recover from your runs.

4. Target Weaknesses and Imbalances: Use cross-training to target weaknesses and imbalances that may arise from repetitive motion in jogging. Incorporate exercises that strengthen and stabilize key muscle groups such as the core, hips, glutes, and upper body to improve overall strength, balance, and injury resilience.

5. Focus on Active Recovery: Use cross-training as a form of active recovery to promote circulation, reduce muscle soreness, and enhance recovery between hard workouts. Engage in low-intensity activities such as cycling, swimming, or foam rolling to flush out metabolic waste products and facilitate recovery.

6. Listen to Your Body: Pay attention to how your body responds to cross-training activities and adjust accordingly. If you experience pain, discomfort, or excessive fatigue, scale back the intensity or duration of your workouts and prioritize rest and recovery as needed.

7. Be Consistent: Incorporate cross-training into your routine on a regular basis to reap the full benefits of diverse physical activity. Aim for a balanced approach that includes a mix of jogging, cross-training, and rest to support overall health, fitness, and longevity in your exercise routine.

STAYING MOTIVATED

Maintaining motivation to stick with your jogging routine can be challenging, especially as you navigate the demands of everyday life and encounter obstacles along the way. However, with the right mindset and strategies, you can stay motivated and committed to your fitness goals.

Here are some tips for staying motivated:

Find Your Why: Take some time to reflect on why you started jogging in the first place. Whether it's to improve your health, boost your energy levels, relieve stress, or challenge yourself, clarifying your reasons for jogging can provide a powerful source of motivation and inspiration.

Set Realistic Goals: Set specific, achievable goals that align with your aspirations and abilities. Break larger goals down into smaller, manageable milestones, and celebrate your progress along the way. Having clear goals to work towards can help keep you focused and motivated, even when faced with obstacles or setbacks.

Mix Up Your Routine: Keep your workouts fresh and exciting by incorporating variety into your jogging routine. Explore new routes, try different types of runs (e.g., intervals, tempo runs, long runs), or incorporate cross-training activities to prevent boredom and keep your workouts engaging.

Find Accountability: Share your goals and progress with a friend, family member, or workout buddy who can provide support, encouragement, and accountability. Knowing that someone else is counting on you can help keep you motivated and accountable to stick with your jogging routine, even on days when you're feeling less motivated.

Track Your Progress: Keep track of your workouts, mileage, pace, and other relevant metrics to monitor your progress over time. Seeing tangible improvements in your performance and fitness can provide a sense of accomplishment and motivation to keep pushing yourself further.

Reward Yourself: Set up a system of rewards to celebrate your achievements and milestones along the way. Whether it's treating yourself to a massage, buying yourself a new piece of workout gear, or indulging in a favorite healthy treat, acknowledging your hard work and dedication can help reinforce positive habits and keep you motivated.

Stay Positive: Cultivate a positive mindset and focus on the benefits and rewards of your jogging routine. Practice gratitude for the opportunity to move your body and improve your health, and remind yourself of the progress you've made and the obstacles you've overcome. Surround yourself with positive influences and affirmations that uplift and inspire you to keep going.

Remember, motivation may ebb and flow, and it's normal to have days when you feel less motivated than others. During these times, draw upon your inner strength, resilience, and commitment to stay focused on your goals and keep moving forward. Staying connected to your why, setting realistic goals, finding accountability, tracking your progress, rewarding yourself, staying positive, and embracing variety, you can stay motivated and committed to your jogging routine at the age of 40 and beyond.

Finding a Running Buddy or Group

Running with a buddy or joining a running group can provide motivation, accountability, and camaraderie, making your jogging routine more enjoyable and rewarding.

Here are some tips for finding a running buddy or group:

1. Reach Out to Friends and Family: Start by reaching out to friends, family members, or coworkers who are interested in jogging or have similar fitness goals. Invite them to join you for a run or suggest forming a running group to support each other's progress and share the experience.

2. Use Social Media and Online Platforms: Explore social media platforms, online forums, and running communities to connect with other runners in your area. Join local running groups or clubs on platforms like Facebook, Meetup, to find like-minded individuals who share your passion for jogging.

3. Check with Local Running Stores: Many local running stores host group runs, training programs, or events for runners of all levels. Check with your nearest running store to see if they offer group runs or if they can connect you with other runners in the community.

4. Attend Park Runs or Community Events: Participate in park runs, charity races, or community events to meet other runners and connect with the local running community. These events provide opportunities to socialize, network, and find potential running buddies or groups to join.

5. Join a Running Club: Consider joining a local running club or organization that offers group runs, training programs, and social events for runners of all abilities. Running clubs provide a supportive and inclusive environment where you can meet new people, improve your running skills, and stay motivated to reach your goals.

6. Use Running Apps: Explore running apps and platforms that connect you with other runners in your area. Apps like Strava, Garmin Connect, and Nike Run Club allow you to find and connect with nearby runners, join virtual challenges, and participate in group activities.

7. Be Open and Approachable: Be open to meeting new people and striking up conversations with fellow runners you encounter on your jogs. Exchange contact information with runners you connect with and suggest meeting up for future runs or workouts.

8. Start Your Own Group: If you're unable to find a suitable running buddy or group in your area, consider starting your own running group. Post flyers at local gyms, parks, or community centers, and use social media to spread the word and attract other runners interested in joining your group.

Setting Short and Long-Term Goals

Setting both short and long-term goals is essential for maintaining motivation, tracking progress, and staying focused on your jogging journey.

Here's how to effectively set and pursue your goals:

Short-Term Goals:

1. Focus on Achievable Milestones: Set short-term goals that are specific, measurable, achievable, relevant, and time-bound (SMART). For example, aim to jog a certain distance or complete a specific workout within the next week or month.

2. Break Larger Goals into Smaller Steps: Break down larger long-term goals into smaller, manageable steps or milestones. This allows you to track progress more easily and maintain momentum as you work towards your larger objectives.

3. Celebrate Small Wins: Celebrate each small achievement along the way to keep yourself motivated and inspired. Acknowledge your progress, whether it's improving your pace, increasing your mileage, or completing a challenging workout.

4. Adapt and Adjust as Needed: Be flexible with your short-term goals and be willing to adjust them based on changing circumstances or feedback from your body. If you encounter setbacks or obstacles,

reassess your goals and adjust your approach as needed to stay on track.

Long-Term Goals:

1. Define Your Ultimate Objectives: Identify your long-term aspirations and ultimate objectives for your jogging journey. Whether it's completing a marathon, improving your overall fitness, or achieving a specific time goal, clarify what success looks like for you in the long term.

2. Set Specific Targets: Set specific and measurable long-term targets that align with your overarching goals. Break down your long-term objectives into smaller, actionable steps that you can work towards over time.

3. Create a Timeline: Establish a realistic timeline for achieving your long-term goals, taking into account factors such as your current fitness level, available time for training, and any potential obstacles or challenges you may encounter along the way.

4. Stay Committed and Consistent: Stay committed to your long-term goals and maintain consistency in your training and lifestyle habits. Consistent effort over time is key to making progress towards your goals and achieving long-term success.

5. Monitor and Evaluate Progress: Regularly monitor your progress towards your long-term goals and evaluate your performance. Keep track of your workouts, mileage, pace, and other relevant metrics to assess your progress and identify areas for improvement.

6. Adjust and Refine Your Approach: Be willing to adjust your long-term goals and modify your approach as needed based on feedback from your body and your progress towards your objectives. Stay adaptable and open to making changes as you learn and grow throughout your jogging journey.

Setting both short and long-term goals that are specific, measurable, achievable, relevant, and time-bound, you can stay motivated, track progress, and work towards achieving your aspirations in your jogging routine at the age of 40 and beyond. Remember to celebrate your successes along the way and stay committed to your journey, even when faced with challenges or setbacks.

Celebrating Milestones

Celebrating milestones is an important part of the jogging journey, as it allows you to acknowledge your progress, stay motivated, and reflect on your achievements.

 Here are some ways to celebrate your jogging milestones:

1. Reflect on Your Progress: Take time to reflect on how far you've come since you started your jogging journey. Celebrate the milestones you've reached, whether it's completing your first 5K, increasing your mileage, improving your pace, or consistently sticking to your workout routine.

2. Reward Yourself: Treat yourself to a reward or indulgence as a way of celebrating your achievements. Whether it's buying yourself a new pair of running shoes, treating yourself to a massage or spa day, or enjoying a favorite meal or treat, find a way to reward yourself for reaching your milestones.

3. Share Your Success: Share your accomplishments with others and celebrate your milestones with friends, family, or fellow runners. Whether it's posting about your achievements on social media, sharing them in a running group or community, or simply telling someone close to you, sharing your success can amplify the joy and satisfaction you feel.

4. Create a Ritual: Establish a special ritual or tradition to mark each milestone you reach in your jogging journey. This could be something simple like taking a post-run selfie at the end of each workout, writing in a journal to reflect on your progress, or treating yourself to a special activity or outing to celebrate your achievements.

5. Set New Goals: Use your milestones as an opportunity to set new goals and challenge yourself to continue progressing in your jogging journey. Whether it's aiming for a new distance or time goal, signing up for a race or event, or focusing on improving your overall fitness, setting new goals keeps you motivated and focused on the next steps in your journey.

6. Practice Gratitude: Take a moment to express gratitude for your health, strength, and the ability to pursue your jogging goals. Cultivate a sense of appreciation for the progress you've made and the opportunities that lie ahead in your jogging journey.

7. Enjoy the Journey: Remember to savor the journey and enjoy the process of pursuing your jogging goals. Celebrate the small victories along the way, embrace the challenges and obstacles you encounter, and find joy and fulfillment in the act of running and pushing yourself to new heights.

DEALING WITH CHALLENGES

Embarking on a jogging journey at the age of 40 comes with its own set of challenges, but with perseverance and resilience, you can overcome obstacles and continue progressing towards your goals. Here are some strategies for dealing with challenges along the way:

1. Embrace the Process: Understand that challenges are a natural part of any journey, including your jogging routine. Instead of viewing obstacles as roadblocks, see them as opportunities for growth and learning. Embrace the process of overcoming challenges and trust that each setback is a chance to become stronger and more resilient.

2. Stay Flexible: Be willing to adapt and adjust your approach in response to challenges or unexpected circumstances. If your schedule changes, the weather doesn't cooperate, or you encounter physical limitations, find alternative solutions or modify your plans to keep moving forward. Flexibility is key to navigating the ups and downs of your jogging journey.

3. Seek Support: Don't hesitate to reach out for support when facing challenges. Whether it's seeking advice from a coach, trainer, or fellow runner, or leaning on friends and family for encouragement, having a support system in place can help you navigate difficult times and stay motivated to overcome obstacles.

4. Practice Self-Compassion: Be kind to yourself and practice self-compassion when facing challenges. Acknowledge that setbacks are a normal part of the journey and that it's okay to experience frustration, disappointment, or self-doubt. Treat yourself with the same kindness and understanding that you would offer to a friend facing similar challenges.

5. Break it Down: Break down challenges into smaller, more manageable steps or tasks. Focus on what you can control and take action one step at a time. By breaking challenges into smaller pieces, they become less daunting and more achievable, allowing you to make progress even in the face of adversity.

6. Stay Positive: Maintain a positive mindset and focus on the solutions rather than dwelling on the problem. Cultivate a sense of optimism and resilience, and remind yourself of your strengths, accomplishments, and past successes. By adopting a positive outlook, you can maintain motivation and momentum even when facing challenges.

7. Learn and Grow: View challenges as opportunities for growth and self-improvement. Reflect on what you can learn from each obstacle you encounter and use it as an opportunity to refine your approach, build resilience, and become a stronger, more capable runner.

Embracing the process, staying flexible, seeking support, practicing self-compassion, breaking challenges down, staying positive, and learning and growing from obstacles, you can navigate challenges with confidence and continue progressing in your jogging journey at the age of 40 and beyond. Remember that resilience is built through overcoming adversity, and each challenge you face makes you stronger and more resilient in the long run.

Weather Conditions

Weather conditions can have a significant impact on your jogging routine, influencing factors such as your comfort, safety, and performance. Whether you're facing hot summer days, chilly winter mornings, or unpredictable weather patterns, it's important to consider how to adapt your workouts accordingly.

In hot and humid conditions, it's essential to stay hydrated and take precautions to prevent heat-related illnesses such as heat exhaustion or heatstroke. Consider jogging during the cooler parts of the day, such as early morning or late evening, to avoid the peak heat hours. Wear lightweight, breathable clothing and a hat or visor to protect yourself from the sun's rays, and apply sunscreen to exposed skin. Listen to your body and adjust your pace or distance as needed to prevent overheating.

During cold weather, layering is key to staying warm and comfortable while jogging. Start with a moisture-wicking base layer to keep sweat away from your skin, add a insulating layer such as a fleece or thermal shirt for warmth, and top it off with a windproof and waterproof outer layer to protect against the elements. Wear gloves, a hat, and thermal leggings or pants to keep extremities warm, and consider investing in reflective gear or a headlamp if jogging in low-light conditions.

In rainy or inclement weather, waterproof and water-resistant gear can help keep you dry and comfortable during your runs. Invest in a waterproof jacket or shell, moisture-wicking socks, and water-resistant shoes to protect yourself from the rain and prevent chafing or blisters. Be cautious of slippery surfaces and adjust your pace or route to avoid hazards such as puddles or slick pavement. Consider using a treadmill or indoor track as an alternative on particularly rainy or stormy days.

In windy conditions, be mindful of wind chill and adjust your clothing layers accordingly to stay warm. Dress in form-fitting layers to minimize wind resistance and consider running into the wind on the outward portion of your route and with the wind at your back on the return leg. Be cautious of gusty winds that may affect your balance or stability, and adjust your pace or route to compensate for the added resistance.

Regardless of the weather conditions, safety should always be a top priority when jogging outdoors. Be aware of your surroundings, stay visible to others by wearing reflective gear or bright colors, and consider carrying a phone or ID in case of emergencies. Listen to weather forecasts and heed any warnings or advisories issued by local authorities to ensure your safety while jogging in various weather conditions.

Time Management

Managing your time effectively is crucial for maintaining a consistent jogging routine, especially when balancing the demands of work, family, and other responsibilities. Here are some tips for managing your time and fitting jogging into your busy schedule:

Prioritize Exercise: Make exercise a priority in your daily schedule by setting aside dedicated time for jogging. Treat your workouts as non-negotiable appointments and commit to sticking to your schedule as much as possible. Consider jogging in the morning before work or in the evening after dinner to avoid conflicts with other obligations.

Plan Ahead: Plan your workouts in advance by scheduling them into your calendar or planner. Consider factors such as weather conditions, time of day, and available daylight when planning your runs, and adjust your schedule accordingly. Having a clear plan in place helps you stay organized and ensures that you make time for exercise each day.

Be Flexible: Be willing to be flexible with your schedule and adapt to changes as needed. Life is unpredictable, and there may be times when unexpected events or obligations arise that disrupt your planned workout time. Instead of getting discouraged, look for alternative opportunities to fit in exercise later in the day or on a different day altogether.

Break it Up: If you're short on time, consider breaking up your workouts into shorter, more manageable sessions throughout the day. For example, you could jog for 15 minutes in the morning before work, take a brisk walk during your lunch break, and finish with a 15-minute jog in the evening. Breaking up your workouts allows you to accumulate exercise throughout the day and makes it easier to fit into a busy schedule.

Combine Activities: Look for opportunities to combine exercise with other activities in your daily routine. For example, you could jog to run errands or commute to work by foot or bicycle instead of driving. Incorporating physical activity into your daily tasks saves time and allows you to multitask while staying active.

Eliminate Time-Wasting Activities: Identify any time-wasting activities or distractions in your daily routine and find ways to eliminate or reduce them. Whether it's scrolling through social media, watching TV, or spending excessive time on non-essential tasks, cutting back on time-wasters frees up more time for exercise and other productive activities.

Set Realistic Expectations: Be realistic about what you can accomplish in a given amount of time and avoid overcommitting yourself. Set manageable goals and prioritize the most important tasks to ensure that you have enough time to devote to exercise without feeling overwhelmed or stressed.

Prioritizing exercise, planning ahead, being flexible, breaking up workouts, combining activities, eliminating time-wasting activities, and setting realistic expectations, you can effectively manage your time and fit jogging into your busy schedule. With dedication and consistency, you can maintain a regular jogging routine and enjoy the many benefits of exercise at the age of 40 and beyond.

Balancing Family and Work Commitments

Balancing family and work commitments while maintaining a jogging routine requires careful planning, communication, and flexibility. Here are some strategies for finding harmony between your personal, professional, and fitness goals:

1. Prioritize Quality Time: Make the most of the time you spend with your family by prioritizing quality over quantity. Allocate dedicated time each day to connect with your loved ones, whether it's during meals, family outings, or shared activities. Be present and engaged during these moments to strengthen your relationships and create lasting memories.

2. Communicate Openly: Keep the lines of communication open with your family members and coworkers to ensure that everyone is on the same page regarding your commitments and priorities. Share your jogging schedule and goals with your family, and discuss how you can work together to support each other's needs and aspirations.

3. Involve Your Family: Find ways to involve your family in your jogging routine and make it a shared experience. Consider inviting your spouse, children, or other family members to join you for a run or participate in a local race or event together. Involving your family in your fitness journey fosters a sense of teamwork and camaraderie while promoting a healthy and active lifestyle for everyone.

4. Plan Family-Friendly Activities: Plan family-friendly activities that accommodate your jogging routine and allow you to spend quality time together. Look for opportunities to combine exercise with family outings, such as hiking, biking, or playing sports at the park. By incorporating physical activity into your family's leisure time, you can promote health and wellness while bonding with your loved ones.

5. Be Flexible with Your Schedule: Be flexible with your jogging schedule and adjust your workouts as needed to accommodate family and work commitments. Consider jogging during off-peak hours, such as early mornings or late evenings, to minimize conflicts with other obligations. Be willing to adapt your schedule based on changing circumstances and prioritize your family's needs when necessary.

6. Set Boundaries: Establish clear boundaries between your work, family, and personal time to prevent burnout and maintain balance in your life. Set aside designated time for work, family, and self-care activities, and avoid allowing one area of your life to encroach on the others. Learn to say no to non-essential commitments and delegate tasks when possible to lighten your load.

7. Practice Self-Care: Prioritize self-care and make time for activities that nourish your mind, body, and soul. Carve out time for relaxation, hobbies, and activities that bring you joy and fulfillment outside of work and family responsibilities. Remember that taking care of yourself allows you to show up as your best self for your loved ones and pursue your fitness goals with renewed energy and enthusiasm.

INJURY PREVENTION AND RECOVERY

Taking proactive steps to prevent injuries and prioritize recovery is essential for maintaining a sustainable jogging routine and avoiding setbacks. Here are some strategies for injury prevention and recovery:

1. Listen to Your Body: Pay attention to any signs or symptoms of discomfort or pain during your runs, and respond accordingly. If you experience pain, discomfort, or unusual fatigue, don't ignore it. Take a break, rest, or seek medical attention if necessary to prevent further injury.

2. Warm Up and Cool Down: Incorporate dynamic warm-up exercises before your runs to prepare your muscles, joints, and cardiovascular system for exercise. Likewise, include a proper cool-down routine after your runs to help reduce muscle soreness and promote recovery.

3. Gradual Progression: Avoid the temptation to increase your mileage, pace, or intensity too quickly, as this can increase the risk of injury. Instead, progress gradually and allow your body time to adapt to increased demands. Follow the 10% rule, which

recommends increasing your mileage or intensity by no more than 10% per week to prevent overuse injuries.

4. Strength Training: Incorporate strength training exercises into your routine to improve muscular strength, endurance, and stability. Focus on exercises that target key muscle groups involved in running, such as the core, hips, glutes, and legs. A strong and balanced musculoskeletal system can help prevent injuries and improve running performance.

5. Cross-Training: Include cross-training activities such as cycling, swimming, or yoga in your routine to provide variety and reduce the risk of overuse injuries. Cross-training allows you to work different muscle groups, improve flexibility, and maintain cardiovascular fitness while giving your body a break from the repetitive impact of running.

6. Proper Footwear: Invest in a good pair of running shoes that provide adequate support, cushioning, and stability for your feet and running gait. Replace your shoes regularly to ensure they continue to provide the necessary protection and shock absorption. Consider consulting with a knowledgeable footwear specialist to find the right shoes for your foot type and running style.

7. Hydration and Nutrition: Stay properly hydrated and fuel your body with nutritious foods to support recovery and reduce the risk of injury. Drink water before, during, and after your runs to maintain hydration, and consume a balanced diet rich in lean protein, complex carbohydrates, healthy fats, vitamins, and minerals. Proper nutrition and hydration are essential for optimal performance and recovery.

8. Rest and Recovery: Make rest and recovery a priority in your training routine to allow your body time to repair and rebuild after workouts. Incorporate rest days into your schedule to prevent overtraining and burnout, and listen to your body's signals for fatigue and fatigue. Practice relaxation techniques such as foam rolling, stretching, yoga, or massage to promote muscle relaxation and reduce tension.

Understanding Common Injuries

Injuries are a common occurrence for runners, but by understanding the types of injuries that can occur and their causes, you can take steps to prevent them and mitigate their impact on your jogging routine.

Here are some common running injuries to be aware of:

1. Shin Splints: Shin splints, or medial tibial stress syndrome, are characterized by pain along the shinbone (tibia) and are often caused by overuse or repetitive stress on the muscles and connective tissues surrounding the shinbone. Contributing factors may include running on hard surfaces, improper footwear, over pronation, or sudden increases in mileage or intensity.

2. Runner's Knee: Runner's knee, or patellofemoral pain syndrome, is a common knee injury characterized by pain around or behind the kneecap (patella). It is often caused by biomechanical imbalances, such as weak hip or quadriceps muscles, improper running form, or overuse. Factors such as running downhill or on uneven terrain can also contribute to runner's knee.

3. IT Band Syndrome: IT band syndrome occurs when the iliotibial (IT) band, a thick band of tissue that runs along the outside of the thigh, becomes inflamed or irritated. This often results in pain on the outside of the knee or hip and can be caused by overuse, tightness

or weakness in the IT band or surrounding muscles, improper running form, or inadequate warm-up or cool-down routines.

4. Plantar Fasciitis: Plantar fasciitis is a common foot injury characterized by pain and inflammation in the plantar fascia, a thick band of tissue that runs along the bottom of the foot. It is often caused by overuse, tight calf muscles, poor foot mechanics, or wearing shoes with inadequate support. Runners with high arches or flat feet may be more susceptible to plantar fasciitis.

5. Achilles Tendonitis: Achilles tendonitis is inflammation of the Achilles tendon, the large tendon that connects the calf muscles to the heel bone. It is often caused by overuse, tight calf muscles, sudden increases in mileage or intensity, or improper footwear. Runners with excessive pronation or a history of calf injuries may be at higher risk for Achilles tendonitis.

6. Stress Fractures: Stress fractures are small cracks or fractures in the bones caused by repetitive stress or overuse. They often occur in the shins (tibia), feet, or hips and are typically associated with sudden increases in training volume, running on hard surfaces, or biomechanical issues such as over pronation or poor running form.

RICE Method (Rest, Ice, Compression, Elevation)

The RICE method is a widely used approach for treating acute injuries and managing pain and inflammation.

It consists of four key components: Rest, Ice, Compression, and Elevation.

Rest: Rest is essential for allowing injured tissues to heal and recover. It involves avoiding activities that exacerbate pain or discomfort and giving the injured area time to rest and recuperate. Depending on the severity of the injury, rest may involve temporarily modifying or reducing physical activity until symptoms improve.

Ice: Applying ice to the injured area helps reduce pain, inflammation, and swelling by constricting blood vessels and numbing the affected area. Ice can be applied using a cold pack, ice pack, or bag of frozen vegetables wrapped in a thin cloth to protect the skin. Apply ice to the injured area for 15-20 minutes at a time, several times a day, especially during the first 48 hours after the injury occurs.

Compression: Compression helps reduce swelling and stabilize the injured area by applying gentle pressure to the surrounding tissues. Compression can be achieved using an elastic bandage or compression wrap applied snugly but not too tightly around the injured area. Ensure that the compression wrap is not too tight, as this can impair circulation and exacerbate swelling.

Elevation: Elevating the injured area above the level of the heart helps reduce swelling and promote drainage of excess fluid from the affected tissues. For example, if the injury is in the lower extremities, elevate the injured leg on a stack of pillows or cushions while lying down or sitting. Aim to keep the injured area elevated as much as possible, especially during periods of rest or sleep.

Using the RICE method, you can effectively manage acute injuries, reduce pain and inflammation, and promote healing and recovery. However, it's important to remember that the RICE method is most effective for treating acute injuries in the early stages and may not be appropriate for all types of injuries or conditions. If you have questions or concerns about the RICE method or your specific injury, consult a healthcare professional for personalized advice and treatment recommendations.

Seeking Professional Help When Necessary

Seeking professional help when necessary is crucial for effectively managing injuries, addressing underlying issues, and promoting optimal recovery. While self-care techniques such as the RICE method can be helpful for managing acute injuries in the short term, certain situations may warrant professional evaluation and treatment.

Here are some signs that indicate it may be time to seek professional help:

Persistent Pain: If you experience persistent or severe pain that does not improve with rest, ice, or over-the-counter pain medications, it may be indicative of a more serious underlying injury or condition. Consulting a healthcare professional can help diagnose the cause of your pain and determine the appropriate treatment plan.

Limited Range of Motion: Difficulty moving the injured area or reduced range of motion may indicate a more severe injury, such as a muscle strain, ligament tear, or joint injury. Seeking evaluation from a healthcare provider can help assess the extent of the injury and guide appropriate rehabilitation efforts.

Swelling or Bruising: Swelling, bruising, or discoloration around the injured area may be signs of inflammation, tissue damage, or internal bleeding. While mild swelling and bruising are common with many injuries, excessive or persistent swelling may warrant further evaluation by a healthcare professional to rule out more serious complications.

Instability or Weakness: Instability, weakness, or feelings of giving way in the injured area may indicate damage to supporting structures such as ligaments or tendons. These symptoms can impair function and increase the risk of further injury if left untreated. A healthcare professional can assess the stability of the injured area and recommend appropriate treatment, such as bracing, physical therapy, or surgery.

Persistent Symptoms: If symptoms persist or worsen over time despite conservative measures, it's important to seek professional evaluation to identify the underlying cause and develop a targeted treatment plan. Ignoring persistent symptoms can lead to chronic pain, functional limitations, and long-term consequences.

Inability to Bear Weight: If you are unable to bear weight on the injured limb or unable to perform daily activities due to pain or instability, it may indicate a more severe injury that requires medical attention. A healthcare professional can perform a thorough evaluation, order diagnostic tests if necessary, and recommend appropriate interventions to facilitate healing and recovery.

JOGGING FOR MENTAL WELL-BEING

Jogging can have significant benefits for mental well-being, providing a natural and accessible way to improve mood, reduce stress, and enhance overall mental health.

Here are some ways jogging can positively impact mental well-being:

1. Stress Reduction: Jogging is a powerful stress reliever, helping to reduce levels of stress hormones such as cortisol and adrenaline while promoting the release of endorphins, the body's natural mood elevators. The rhythmic movement of jogging, combined with being outdoors in nature, can have a calming effect on the mind and help alleviate feelings of tension and anxiety.

2. Mood Enhancement: Regular jogging has been shown to improve mood and emotional well-being by increasing levels of serotonin and dopamine, neurotransmitters associated with feelings of happiness and pleasure. Engaging in physical activity releases these "feel-good" chemicals in the brain, leading to a sense of euphoria and satisfaction.

3. Anxiety Management: Jogging can be an effective way to manage symptoms of anxiety and promote relaxation. The repetitive motion of jogging can serve as a form of meditation in motion, allowing individuals to focus their attention on the present moment and quiet the mind. Additionally, the sense of accomplishment and empowerment that comes from completing a jog can boost confidence and self-esteem.

4. Cognitive Benefits: Jogging has cognitive benefits as well, improving cognitive function, concentration, and memory. Regular aerobic exercise has been shown to stimulate the growth of new brain cells and enhance brain plasticity, leading to improved cognitive performance and overall brain health.

5. Sleep Improvement: Engaging in regular exercise such as jogging can improve sleep quality and duration, which is essential for overall mental well-being. Physical activity helps regulate sleep patterns, making it easier to fall asleep and stay asleep throughout the night. Adequate sleep is crucial for mental clarity, emotional resilience, and stress management.

6. Social Connection: Jogging can provide opportunities for social interaction and connection, whether through joining a running group, participating in local races or events, or simply jogging with friends or family members. Social support and companionship can

enhance feelings of belongingness and reduce feelings of loneliness or isolation, contributing to overall mental well-being.

7. Self-Care and Mindfulness: Incorporating jogging into your routine can serve as a form of self-care and mindfulness, allowing you to prioritize your physical and mental health. Taking time for yourself to engage in a jog can be a valuable opportunity to disconnect from stressors, reconnect with yourself, and cultivate a sense of balance and well-being.

Jogging offers a holistic approach to mental well-being, providing physical exercise, stress relief, mood enhancement, cognitive benefits, social connection, and opportunities for self-care and mindfulness. By incorporating jogging into your routine regularly, you can reap the many mental health benefits and improve your overall quality of life.

Stress Reduction Benefits

Jogging offers numerous benefits for stress reduction, providing a natural and effective way to alleviate tension, unwind, and promote relaxation. Here are some of the stress reduction benefits of jogging:

1. Stress Hormone Regulation: Jogging helps regulate the body's stress response by reducing levels of stress hormones such as cortisol and adrenaline. Cortisol is often referred to as the "stress hormone" because its levels increase in response to stressors, contributing to feelings of tension and anxiety. Engaging in physical activity like jogging can lower cortisol levels, helping to alleviate stress and promote a sense of calm.

2. Endorphin Release: Jogging stimulates the release of endorphins, the body's natural painkillers and mood elevators. Endorphins are neurotransmitters that interact with the brain's receptors to reduce feelings of pain and produce feelings of pleasure and euphoria. The "runner's high" experienced during and after jogging is attributed to the release of endorphins, which can help alleviate stress and improve mood.

3. Muscle Relaxation: The repetitive motion of jogging can help relax tense muscles and relieve physical tension built up during periods of stress. As you jog, your muscles contract and release rhythmically, promoting blood flow and oxygenation to muscle

tissues. This increased circulation can help loosen tight muscles, reduce muscle stiffness, and alleviate physical discomfort associated with stress.

4. Mental Distraction: Jogging provides a mental distraction from stressors and worries, allowing you to focus your attention on the present moment and the physical sensations of running. The rhythmic motion of jogging can be meditative, helping to quiet the mind and temporarily shift your focus away from stress-inducing thoughts. Many people find that jogging serves as a form of "moving meditation," promoting mindfulness and relaxation.

5. Improved Sleep Quality: Regular jogging can improve sleep quality and duration, which is essential for stress reduction and overall well-being. Physical activity helps regulate sleep patterns by promoting deeper, more restorative sleep and reducing the incidence of sleep disturbances. Better sleep quality can help lower stress levels, enhance mood, and improve cognitive function during waking hours.

6. Sense of Accomplishment: Completing a jog, whether it's a short run around the block or a longer distance run, can instill a sense of accomplishment and empowerment. Setting and achieving fitness goals through jogging can boost self-esteem, confidence, and resilience, which can help mitigate the impact of stressors in other areas of life.

Mindfulness Practices While Jogging

Practicing mindfulness while jogging can enhance your overall experience and deepen the benefits of your run. Here are some mindfulness practices you can incorporate into your jogging routine:

1. Focus on the Present Moment: Bring your attention to the present moment by tuning in to the sensations of your body as you jog. Notice the rhythm of your breath, the feeling of your feet striking the ground, and the movement of your muscles. Let go of distractions and worries about the past or future, and immerse yourself fully in the present experience of running.

2. Practice Breath Awareness: Pay attention to your breath as you jog, using it as an anchor to keep you grounded in the present moment. Notice the sensation of air flowing in and out of your lungs, the rise and fall of your chest, and the rhythm of your breath as you move. Focusing on your breath can help calm the mind, reduce stress, and promote relaxation.

3. Observe Your Surroundings: Take time to notice and appreciate the sights, sounds, and sensations of your environment as you jog. Notice the colors of the sky, the sounds of nature, and the feeling of the breeze on your skin. Cultivate a sense of curiosity and wonder as you explore your surroundings, allowing yourself to be fully present and engaged in the moment.

4. Practice Body Scan Meditation: Conduct a body scan meditation while jogging, systematically bringing awareness to different parts of your body from head to toe. Notice any areas of tension, discomfort, or fatigue, and consciously release tension as you continue to jog. Pay attention to how your body feels as you move, and make any necessary adjustments to improve your posture or stride.

5. Practice Gratitude: Cultivate an attitude of gratitude as you jog by reflecting on the things you are grateful for in your life. Express gratitude for your health, the opportunity to move your body, and the beauty of nature surrounding you. Focusing on gratitude can shift your perspective from stress and negativity to positivity and appreciation.

6. Set Intentions: Set positive intentions for your jog, such as focusing on joy, vitality, or inner peace. Visualize yourself achieving your goals and embodying the qualities you wish to cultivate during your run. Setting intentions can help guide your mindset and energy throughout your jog, empowering you to make the most of the experience.

Incorporating Jogging into Your Self-Care Routine

Incorporating jogging into your self-care routine can be a powerful way to prioritize your physical and mental well-being and enhance your overall quality of life.

Here's how jogging can become an integral part of your self-care regimen:

Mind-Body Connection: Jogging provides an opportunity to connect with your body and cultivate awareness of physical sensations, breath, and movement. By tuning into your body's signals and needs during your run, you can develop a deeper understanding of yourself and promote mind-body harmony.

Stress Relief: Jogging is an effective stress reliever, helping to reduce levels of stress hormones and promote relaxation. Taking time out of your day to go for a jog can provide a much-needed break from the demands of work, family, and other responsibilities, allowing you to clear your mind, release tension, and recharge your batteries.

Mental Clarity: Jogging can enhance mental clarity and focus by providing a break from the constant stream of thoughts and distractions. The rhythmic movement of jogging and the meditative quality of being in motion can help quiet the mind, improve concentration, and promote mental clarity.

Emotional Well-Being: Regular jogging can have a positive impact on emotional well-being, helping to improve mood, reduce symptoms of anxiety and depression, and boost self-esteem. The release of endorphins during exercise promotes feelings of happiness and contentment, while the sense of accomplishment that comes from completing a run can boost confidence and self-efficacy.

Self-Reflection: Jogging offers a chance for self-reflection and introspection, allowing you to process thoughts and emotions in a supportive and non-judgmental environment. Use your time on the road or trail to reflect on your goals, values, and priorities, and consider how you can align your actions with your intentions for a more fulfilling life.

Connection to Nature: Jogging outdoors allows you to connect with the natural world and appreciate the beauty of your surroundings. Spending time in nature has been shown to reduce stress, improve mood, and enhance overall well-being, making outdoor jogging a nourishing experience for both body and soul.

Personal Growth: Incorporating jogging into your self-care routine can facilitate personal growth and development by challenging you to push past your comfort zone, set and achieve goals, and overcome obstacles. Each run presents an opportunity for growth and self-discovery, helping you build resilience, confidence, and a sense of empowerment.

Integrating jogging into your self-care routine, you can reap the myriad benefits for your physical, mental, and emotional well-being. Whether you jog for stress relief, mental clarity, emotional balance, or personal growth, prioritizing regular exercise can be a powerful form of self-care that nourishes your mind, body, and spirit.

CONTINUING YOUR JOURNEY

Continuing your journey with jogging involves embracing the ongoing process of growth, learning, and self-discovery as you strive to maintain a sustainable and fulfilling running routine. Here are some ways to continue your journey with jogging:

1. Set New Goals: Keep your jogging routine fresh and exciting by setting new goals to work towards. Whether it's increasing your mileage, improving your pace, or training for a specific race or event, having goals gives you something to strive for and helps keep you motivated and focused.

2. Explore New Routes: Break out of your routine by exploring new running routes and environments. Seek out scenic trails, urban paths, or local parks to add variety to your runs and keep things interesting. Exploring new routes can invigorate your workouts and inspire a sense of adventure and exploration.

3. Mix Up Your Workouts: Incorporate variety into your jogging routine by mixing up your workouts with different types of runs and cross-training activities. Try interval training, hill repeats, tempo runs, or fartlek workouts to challenge yourself and improve your fitness level. Cross-training activities such as cycling, swimming, or strength training can complement your running routine and prevent burnout.

4. Listen to Your Body: Pay attention to your body's signals and adjust your jogging routine accordingly. Be mindful of any signs of fatigue, pain, or overtraining, and give yourself permission to rest and recover when needed. Prioritize self-care and listen to your body's needs to avoid injury and maintain long-term sustainability.

5. Connect with Others: Cultivate a sense of community and support by connecting with other runners. Join a local running group, participate in online forums or social media groups, or find a running buddy to share your experiences and challenges with. Surrounding yourself with like-minded individuals can provide motivation, accountability, and encouragement on your jogging journey.

6. Reflect and Celebrate: Take time to reflect on your progress and celebrate your achievements along the way. Acknowledge the hard work and dedication you've put into your jogging routine and celebrate milestones, whether it's reaching a new distance, setting a personal record, or simply enjoying a satisfying run. Celebrating your successes helps reinforce your commitment to your jogging journey and fuels your motivation to continue moving forward.

7. Embrace the Journey: Above all, embrace the journey of jogging as a lifelong pursuit of health, happiness, and personal growth. Recognize that progress is not always linear and that setbacks and challenges are a natural part of the process. Approach each run with curiosity, gratitude, and an open heart, and allow yourself to fully experience the joys and rewards of being a runner.

Progression Beyond Beginner Levels

Progressing beyond beginner levels in jogging involves building upon your foundation of fitness, endurance, and experience to challenge yourself and reach new heights in your running journey.

Here are some strategies for advancing your skills and performance as a runner:

1. Gradual Increase in Mileage: As you become more comfortable with jogging, gradually increase your mileage to build endurance and improve your aerobic capacity. Focus on adding distance to your runs gradually, increasing your weekly mileage by no more than 10% to avoid overuse injuries and allow your body time to adapt.

2. Incorporate Speed Work: Introduce speed work into your training routine to improve your running speed and efficiency. Interval

training, tempo runs, and fartlek workouts can help you develop your anaerobic capacity, increase your lactate threshold, and enhance your overall performance. Start with shorter intervals and gradually increase the intensity and duration as you become stronger and more experienced.

3. Strength Training: Incorporate strength training exercises into your routine to build muscle strength, power, and resilience. Focus on exercises that target key muscle groups used in running, such as the core, hips, glutes, and legs. Strength training can help improve running economy, reduce the risk of injury, and enhance overall performance.

4. Hill Training: Incorporate hill training into your workouts to improve leg strength, power, and endurance. Running uphill challenges your muscles, cardiovascular system, and mental toughness, while downhill running helps improve eccentric muscle strength and control. Incorporate hills into your regular runs or dedicate specific workouts to hill repeats to reap the benefits of this challenging terrain.

5. Long Runs: Incorporate longer runs into your training routine to build endurance and mental toughness for longer distances. Gradually increase the duration of your long runs to simulate the demands of your target race distance and improve your ability to

sustain effort over time. Long runs also provide an opportunity to practice fueling and hydration strategies for longer races.

6. Recovery and Rest: Prioritize recovery and rest as you increase the intensity and volume of your training. Allow your body time to recover between hard workouts, and listen to your body's signals for fatigue, soreness, or overtraining. Incorporate rest days into your weekly schedule to prevent burnout and promote optimal recovery and adaptation.

7. Race Preparation: If you're interested in participating in races, consider incorporating race-specific workouts into your training plan to prepare for the demands of competition. Practice running at your goal race pace, simulate race conditions in training runs, and develop a race-day strategy to optimize your performance on race day.

8. Consistency and Patience: Remember that progress takes time and consistency, so be patient with yourself as you work towards your goals. Focus on gradual improvement and celebrate your achievements along the way, whether it's completing a new distance, setting a personal record, or simply enjoying the journey as a runner.

Exploring Different Terrain and Routes

Exploring different terrain and routes can breathe new life into your jogging routine, offering fresh challenges, scenery, and experiences that can invigorate your runs and keep you motivated. Here are some reasons to venture beyond your usual jogging routes and explore new terrain:

Variety and Excitement: Running the same route day after day can become monotonous and uninspiring. Exploring different terrain and routes introduces variety and excitement into your jogging routine, keeping things interesting and engaging. Whether it's running through scenic parks, along tranquil waterfronts, or on rugged trails, each new route offers a unique experience and adventure.

Physical Challenges: Different terrains present different physical challenges that can test your strength, endurance, and agility as a runner. Running on hills or trails requires greater muscular effort and coordination than running on flat pavement, challenging your cardiovascular system and improving your overall fitness level. Embracing these challenges can make you a stronger and more well-rounded runner.

Mental Stimulation: Exploring new terrain stimulates your mind and engages your senses in ways that running familiar routes cannot. Taking in new sights, sounds, and smells as you run can be mentally invigorating and refreshing, providing a welcome distraction from the stresses of daily life. Running in nature, in particular, can promote feelings of calm, tranquility, and connectedness to the world around you.

Skill Development: Running on different terrains and surfaces can help you develop new skills and techniques as a runner. Trail running, for example, requires greater focus and attention to foot placement to navigate uneven terrain and obstacles safely. Running on sand or gravel challenges your balance and stability, while running on pavement or track allows you to focus on speed and pacing.

Injury Prevention: Varying your running terrain can help prevent overuse injuries by reducing repetitive stress on the same muscles and joints. Running on softer surfaces such as trails or grass absorbs impact more effectively than running on hard pavement, reducing the strain on your muscles and bones. Mixing in different terrains and surfaces also helps strengthen stabilizing muscles and improve proprioception, reducing the risk of injury over time.

Exploration and Adventure: Above all, exploring different terrain and routes adds an element of exploration and adventure to your jogging routine. Each new route offers the opportunity to discover hidden gems, secret trails, and breathtaking vistas that you may never have encountered otherwise. Embrace the sense of curiosity and wonder that comes with exploring new places, and allow yourself to be open to unexpected surprises and discoveries along the way.

Stepping outside your comfort zone and exploring different terrain and routes, you can enrich your jogging experience, challenge yourself physically and mentally, and cultivate a deeper appreciation for the joys of running. Whether you're running through urban streets, scenic trails, or rugged mountainsides, each new route offers a chance to embrace the freedom, exhilaration, and sense of adventure that comes with being a runner.

Participating in Running Events

Participating in running events can be a rewarding and fulfilling experience that adds excitement, motivation, and camaraderie to your jogging journey. Whether you're a seasoned runner or just starting out, here are some reasons to consider participating in running events:

1. Goal Setting: Running events provide a tangible goal to work towards, whether it's completing a certain distance, achieving a personal best time, or simply crossing the finish line. Setting a goal gives you something to strive for and helps keep you motivated and focused during training.

2. Sense of Accomplishment: Crossing the finish line of a running event is a powerful and gratifying experience that instills a sense of accomplishment and pride. The sense of achievement that comes from completing a race can boost your confidence, self-esteem, and belief in your abilities as a runner.

3. Community and Camaraderie: Running events bring together people of all ages, backgrounds, and abilities who share a common passion for running. Participating in races allows you to connect with fellow runners, share experiences, and form friendships that can last a lifetime. The sense of camaraderie and support among participants creates a supportive and uplifting atmosphere that can enhance your overall running experience.

4. Motivation and Inspiration: Being surrounded by other runners who are pushing their limits and striving towards their goals can be incredibly motivating and inspiring. Seeing others achieve their goals can inspire you to push harder, dig deeper, and overcome your own challenges. The energy and enthusiasm of race day can fuel your determination and help you perform at your best.

5. Sense of Adventure: Running events offer the opportunity to explore new places and experience the thrill of running in different settings and environments. Whether it's running through city streets, scenic parks, or rugged trails, each race presents a new adventure and an opportunity to discover new sights and experiences.

6. Support and Encouragement: Running events provide a supportive and encouraging environment where participants cheer each other on and celebrate each other's accomplishments. The encouragement of spectators, volunteers, and fellow runners can give you an extra boost of energy and motivation when you need it most.

7. Personal Growth: Participating in running events can foster personal growth and development by challenging you to push past your comfort zone, overcome obstacles, and discover your true potential as a runner. Each race presents an opportunity for growth, learning, and self-discovery that can enrich your life both on and off the road.

CONCLUSION

In conclusion, embarking on a journey into the world of jogging at the age of 40 or beyond is not just about improving physical fitness—it's about embracing a lifestyle that nurtures both body and mind. From the initial steps of understanding the benefits of jogging to the exploration of different terrains, setting goals, and participating in running events, the journey is rich with opportunities for growth, self-discovery, and personal fulfillment.

Through this guide, we've explored the importance of overcoming age-related obstacles, assessing your current fitness level, understanding physical limitations, and setting realistic goals. We've delved into the practical aspects of getting the right gear, choosing the right shoes, and creating a jogging plan that works for you. We've also discussed the importance of rest, proper nutrition, hydration, and injury prevention, as well as the significance of mindfulness practices, listening to your body, and seeking professional help when necessary.

As you continue your journey into jogging, remember that progress takes time, patience, and consistency. Embrace the process, celebrate your successes, and learn from setbacks along the way. Whether you're jogging for stress relief, mental clarity, physical health, or simply the joy of movement, know that every step you take is a step towards a happier, healthier, and more vibrant life.

Above all, cherish the journey itself—the exhilarating rush of wind against your face, the rhythmic pounding of your feet on the pavement, the quiet moments of reflection and introspection as you run. Embrace the sense of freedom, empowerment, and connection that comes with being a runner, and allow yourself to fully experience the transformative power of jogging in all its forms.

So lace up your shoes, hit the road, and embrace the journey that lies ahead. With determination, perseverance, and a willingness to explore, the possibilities are endless. Here's to a lifetime of joyful, fulfilling, and meaningful experiences on the open road of jogging. **Happy running!**

Reflecting on Your Journey

Reflecting on your journey into jogging can be a valuable opportunity to celebrate your progress, learn from your experiences, and set new intentions for the future. Take a moment to pause and consider how far you've come since you first laced up your running shoes. Reflect on the highs and lows, the challenges you've overcome, and the lessons you've learned along the way.

Consider the physical gains you've achieved—the increased endurance, strength, and stamina that have come with consistent training. Celebrate the milestones you've reached—the first mile you ran without stopping, the personal records you set in races, or the distances you never thought possible. Acknowledge the dedication and commitment it took to stick with your jogging routine, even on days when motivation was lacking or obstacles seemed insurmountable.

But don't just focus on the physical aspects of your journey—take time to reflect on the mental and emotional benefits as well. Consider how jogging has improved your mood, reduced stress, and brought a sense of peace and clarity to your life. Reflect on the moments of joy, exhilaration, and profound connection with yourself and the world around you that running has provided.

As you reflect on your journey, also consider the challenges you've faced—the injuries, setbacks, and moments of doubt that tested your resolve. Reflect on how you navigated these challenges with resilience, perseverance, and determination, and consider what you learned about yourself in the process. Use these experiences as opportunities for growth and self-discovery, knowing that setbacks are often the stepping stones to greater success.

Looking ahead, consider what you want to achieve in your jogging journey moving forward. Set new goals that challenge and inspire you, whether it's completing a longer distance, improving your pace, or exploring new trails and terrain. Reflect on how you can continue to prioritize self-care, listen to your body, and cultivate mindfulness and gratitude in your running practice.

Above all, remember to savor the journey itself—the sights, sounds, and sensations of each run, the friendships forged along the way, and the profound sense of freedom and empowerment that comes with being a runner. Embrace the ups and downs, the triumphs and setbacks, knowing that each step you take is a part of your unique and unfolding journey into the transformative world of jogging.

Encouragement for Sustained Commitment

For those embarking on a jogging journey, sustaining commitment is essential for long-term success.

Here's some encouragement to help you stay committed:

1. Celebrate Progress: Take pride in every milestone, whether it's completing a challenging run, setting a new personal record, or simply showing up and lacing up your shoes. Celebrate your progress and acknowledge the hard work and dedication it took to get there.

2. Embrace Setbacks: Remember that setbacks are a natural part of any journey, including your jogging journey. Instead of letting setbacks discourage you, use them as opportunities for growth and learning. Stay resilient, stay focused, and keep moving forward.

3. Find Your Why: Remind yourself why you started jogging in the first place and reconnect with your reasons for wanting to improve your health and well-being. Whether it's to reduce stress, boost mood, or achieve a specific fitness goal, keep your "why" front and center to help sustain your commitment.

4. Set Realistic Goals: Break down your long-term goals into smaller, manageable steps and set realistic expectations for yourself.

Celebrate progress along the way and adjust your goals as needed to stay motivated and on track.

5. Create Accountability: Surround yourself with a supportive community of friends, family, or fellow runners who can help hold you accountable to your goals. Share your progress, celebrate your achievements, and lean on others for encouragement and support during challenging times.

6. Focus on Consistency: Consistency is key when it comes to sustaining commitment to jogging. Make it a priority to show up and run regularly, even on days when you don't feel like it. Remember that small, consistent efforts add up over time and lead to lasting results.

7. Practice Self-Compassion: Be kind to yourself and practice self-compassion, especially during moments of struggle or setback. Recognize that it's okay to have off days or to fall short of your goals occasionally. Treat yourself with the same kindness and understanding that you would offer to a friend.

8. Mix it Up: Keep your jogging routine fresh and exciting by mixing up your workouts, trying new routes, and exploring different terrains. Incorporate variety into your routine to prevent boredom and burnout and keep your enthusiasm for jogging alive.

9. Visualize Success: Take a moment each day to visualize yourself achieving your goals and envisioning the positive impact that jogging will have on your life. Use visualization techniques to stay focused, motivated, and inspired to continue pushing forward.

10. Stay Positive: Maintain a positive mindset and cultivate an attitude of gratitude for the opportunity to move your body and improve your health through jogging. Focus on the joy and fulfillment that running brings to your life, and let that positivity fuel your commitment to your jogging journey.

Remember that sustained commitment to jogging is not about perfection—it's about progress, growth, and resilience. Stay focused on your goals, stay true to yourself, and keep putting one foot in front of the other, knowing that every step you take brings you closer to becoming the best version of yourself. You've got this!

Final Tips for Long-Term Jogging Success

As you continue your journey into long-term jogging success, here are some final tips to keep in mind:

1. Listen to Your Body: Pay attention to your body's signals and adjust your training accordingly. Rest when you need it, and don't ignore signs of fatigue or injury. Prioritize recovery and self-care to maintain your health and well-being.

2. Stay Flexible: Be willing to adapt and adjust your jogging routine as needed. Life can be unpredictable, so be flexible with your schedule and workouts. Don't be afraid to modify your goals or plans if circumstances change.

3. Practice Patience: Progress in jogging takes time, so be patient with yourself and trust the process. Don't get discouraged by setbacks or slow progress. Stay consistent, stay focused, and keep moving forward one step at a time.

4. Enjoy the Journey: Remember to have fun and enjoy the journey of jogging. Find joy in the process of running, whether it's the feeling of the wind in your hair, the satisfaction of completing a challenging workout, or the camaraderie of running with friends.

5. Stay Inspired: Keep yourself motivated and inspired by setting new goals, trying new routes, and seeking out new challenges. Surround yourself with positive influences, whether it's fellow runners, inspiring books, or uplifting music and podcasts.

6. Stay Safe: Prioritize safety when jogging, especially when running outdoors. Wear reflective clothing, stay hydrated, and be aware of your surroundings. Consider carrying a phone or letting someone know your route and expected return time.

7. Celebrate Successes: Take time to celebrate your achievements and milestones along the way. Whether it's completing a race, reaching a new distance, or simply sticking to your jogging routine, acknowledge your accomplishments and give yourself credit for your hard work.

8. Keep Learning: Continuously seek out opportunities to learn and grow as a runner. Stay informed about training techniques, nutrition strategies, injury prevention, and other aspects of running. Stay open to trying new things and experimenting with different approaches to improve your jogging experience.

9. Give Back: Consider giving back to the running community by volunteering at races, coaching beginner runners, or supporting local running events. Sharing your knowledge and experience can be rewarding and help inspire others on their own jogging journeys.

10. Remember Why You Started: Finally, always remember the reasons why you started jogging in the first place. Whether it's to improve your health, relieve stress, or simply enjoy the freedom of movement, keep your motivations front and center to stay connected to your passion for running.

With these final tips in mind, may you continue to enjoy the many benefits of jogging and experience long-term success and fulfillment on your running journey.

Happy jogging!!!!

www.ingramcontent.com/pod-product-compliance
Lightning Source LLC
Chambersburg PA
CBHW070843250726
48662CB00003B/1347